TRADITIONAL CHINESE TREATMENT FOR HYPERTENSION

Editor in Chief   Hou Jinglun

Associate Editor in Chief   Ren Wuxian

Editors   Li Fulin   Lin Qi

           Li Guohua   Liu Jianxin

Academy Press [Xue Yuan]

First Edition 1995

ISBN7-5077-0996-5/R · 165

TRADITIONAL CHINESE
TREATMENT FOR HYPERTENSION

Editor in Chief   Hou Jinglun

Associate Editor in Chief   Ren Wuxian

Editor   Li Fulin   Lin Qi   Li Guohua   Liu Jianxin

Published by Academy Press [Xue Yuan]

Distributed by

China International Book Trading Corporation

35 Chegongzhuang Xilu, Beijing 100044, China

P. O. Box 399, Beijing, China

Printed in the People's Republic of China

Résumé

Hypertension is commonly seen in the clinic. About 300 million people suffer from hypertension and its complications. It may develop and cause dysfunction and organic changes of brain, heart, and kidneys, etc. , and do great harm to people's health. Up to now, favorable and radical treatment has not been found out in modern medicine. Patients with hypertension have to take medicine for a long period of time or even in all their lives.

Traditional Chinese Medicine (TCM) therapy has gentle and stable effects on hypertension. It may improve the symptoms, reduce the complications, reverse the impairment of target organs, and improve the prognosis. The book consists of 9 chapters. Some knowledge of hypertension in modern medicine is considered briefly in order to help the combination of the

Chinese traditional and Western medicine. This is included in Chapter 1. In Chapter 2, we have discussed TCM knowledge of hypertension — its causes and mechanisms, the differentiation and therapeutic principles and the corresponding recipes. In Chapter 3, varied Chinese herbal medicines are recommended for hypertension. Chapter 4, prescriptions of TCM for lowering blood pressure. In the subsequent 5 chapters, acupuncture treatment, massage therapy, qigong and medicated diet are considered. Nursing care is included in Chapter 9. We have tried to ensure that this book in accurate, practical, and up to date.

Hou Jinglun
Dec. 12,1994

Contents

4

Chapter Three Materia Medica for lowering blood pressure .... (141)

5

Chapter One
HYPERTENSION IN MODERN MEDICINE

Section 1
Hyperiensive vascular disease

An elevated arterial pressure is probably the more important public health problem in developed countries — —being common, asymptomatic, readily detectable, usually easily treatable, and often leading to lethal complications if left untreated. Although our understanding of the pathophysiology of an elevated arterial pressure has increased, in 90 to 95 percent of cases the etiology (and thus potentially the prevention or cure)is still unknown.

1. Definetion

Since there is no dividing line between normal and high blood pressure but also systolic pressure,age, sex, and race. For example, patients with a diastolic pressure greater than 12. 0 kPa (90 mmHg) will have a significant reduction in morbidity and mortality with adequate therapy. These , then, are patients who have hypertension and who should be considered for treatment.

The level of systolic pressure is important in assessing arterial pressure's influence on cardiovascular morbidity. Males with normal diastolic pressures ($<$ 10. 9kPa, 82mmHg) but elevated systolic pressures ($>$21kPa, 158mmHg)have a 2. 5 fold increase in their cardiovascular mortality rates when compared with individuals with similar diastolic pressures but whose systolic pressures are normal($<$17. 3kPa,130mmHg).

Other significant factors which modify blood pressure's influence on the frequency of morbid cardivascular events are age, race, and sex with young black males being most adversely affected by hypertension.

Thus, even though in an adult hypertension is usually defined as a pressure greater than or equal to 150/90mmHg, in men under 45 years of age a pressure greater than or equal to 130/90mmHg may be elevated.

Individuals can be classified as being normotensive

if arterial pressure is less than the levels noted above and as having sustained hypertension if the diastolic pressure always exceeds these levels. Arterial pressure fluctuated in most persons, whether they are normotensive or hypertensive. Those who are classified as having labile hypertension are patients who sometimes but not always have arterial pressures within the hypertensive range. These patients are often considered to have borderline hypertension.

Sustained hypertension can become accelerated or enter a malignant phase. Though a patient with malignant hypertension often has a blood pressure above 200/140mmHg, it is papilledema, usually accompanied by retinal hemorrhages and exudates, and not the absolute pressure level, that defines this condition. Accelerated hypertension signifies a significant recent increase over previous hypertensive levels associated with evidence of vascular damage on funduscopic examination but without papilledema.

In 1978, World health Organization (WHO)determined:

1) Normal blood pressure: Systolic pressure ≤18. 62kPa(140mmHg), diastolic ≤ 12. 0kPa(90mmHg)

2) Hypertension: Systolic pressure ≥ 21. 3kPa

(160mmHg)or diastolic≥12. 6kPa(95mmHg).

3) Borderline hypertension: Systolic pressure 18. 75 ~ 21. 2kPa(141 ~ 159mmHg), diastolic preseure 12. 1~12. 5kPa(91~94mmHg)

2. Etiology

The cause of elevated arterial pressure is unknown in most cases. There are no available data to define the frequency of secondary hypertension in the general population, although in middle-aged males it has been reported to be 6 percent. On the other hand ', in referral centers where patients undergo an extensive evaluation, it has been reported to be as high as 35 percent.

ESSENTIAL HYPERTENSION Patients with arterial hypertension and no definable cause are said to have primary, essential, or idiopathic hypertension. By definition, the underlying mechanism (s) is unknown; however, the kidney probably plays a central role.

Heredity Genetic factors have long been assumed to be important in the genesis of hypertension. One approach has been to assess the correlation of blood pressures within families (familial aggregation). From

4

these studies the minimum size of the genetic factor can be expressed by a correlation coefficient of approximately 0. 2.

Enviromnent   A number of environmental factors have been specifically implicated in the development of hypertension including 9 salt intake, obesity, occupation, family size, and crowding. These factors have all been assumed to be important in the increase in blood pressure with age in more affluent societies, in contrast to the decline in blood pressure with age in more primitive cultures. Indeed, even the familial aggregation of blood pressure has been suggested as being related, at least in part, to environmental rather than genetic factors. However, since adopted children do not demonstrate familial aggregation of blood pressure, this phenomenon is probably almost entirely the result of genetic factors.

Factors modifying the course of essential hypertension Age, race, sex, smoking, serum cholesterol, glucose intolerance, weight, and perhaps renin activity may all alter the prognosis of this disease.

SECONDARY HYPERTENSION   In only a small minority of patients with an elevated arterial pressure can a specific cause be identified. Nearly all the secondary forms are related to an alteration in hormone secretion and or renal function.

Renal hypertension　Hypertension produced by renal disease is the result of either (1) a derangement in the renal handling of sodium and fluids leading to volume expansion or (2) an alteration in renal secretion of vasoactive materials resulting in a systemic or local change in arteriolar tone. A simple explanation for renal vascular hypertension is the decreased perfusion of renal tissue due to stenosis of a main or branch renal artery activated the renin-angiotensin system. The angiotensin elebates arterial pressure by direct vasoconstriction, by stimulation of aldosterone secretion with resultant sodium retention, and/or by stimulating the adrenergic nervous system. In actual practice only about one-half of patients with renovascular hypertension have elevated absolute levels of renin activity in peripheral plasma, although when renin measurements are referenced against an index of sodium balance, a much higher fraction have inappropriately high values.

A recently described form of renal hypertension results from the excess secretion of renin by juxtaglomerular cell tumors or nephroblastyomas. The initial presentation has been similar to that of hyperaldos-

6

teronism with hypertension hypokalemia, and overproduction of aldosterone. However, in contrast to primary aldosteronism, peripheral renin activity is elevated instead of subnormal. This disease can be distinguished from other forms of secondary aldosteronism by the presence of normal renal function and with unilateral increases in renal vein renin concentration without a renal artery lesion.

Endocrine hypertension   Adrenal hypertension is a feature of a variety of adrenal cortical abnormalities. In primary aldosteronism there is a clear relationship between the aldosterone-induced, sodium retention and the hypertension. Normal individuals given aldosterone develop hypertension only if they also ingest sodium. Since aldosterone causes sodium retention by stimulating renal tubular exchange of sodium for potassium, hypokalemia is a prominent feature in most patients with primary aldosteronism, and the measurement of serum potassium provides a simple screening test. The effect of sodium retention and volume expansion in chronically suppressing plasma renin activity is critically important for the definitive diagnosis. In most clinical situations plasma renin activity and plasma or urinary aldosterone levels parallel each other, but in patients with primary aldosteronism, aldosterone levels are high and relatively fixed because of autonomous aldosterone secretion, while plasma renin activity levels are suppressed and respond sluggishly to sodium depletion. Primary aldosteronism may be secondary either to a tumor or bilateral adrenal hyperplasia. It is important to distinguish between two conditions preoperatively, as usually the hypertension in the latter is not modified by operation.

The most common cause of endocrine hypertension is that resulting from the use of estrogen-containing oral contraceptives. Indeed, this may be the most common form of secondary hypertension. The mechanism producing the hypertension is likely to be secondary to activation of the renin-angiotensin-aldosterone system.

Coarctation of the aorta   The hypertension associated with coarctation may be caused by the constriction itaelf, or perhaps by the changes in the renal circulation which result in an unusual form of renal arterial hypertension. The diagnosis of coarctation is usually evident from physical examination and routine x-ray findings.

Low-renin essential hypertension   Approximately 20 percent of patients who by all other criteria have essential hypertension have suppressed plasma renin activity. Recent studies have suggested that many of these patients have an increased sensitivity to angiotensin II which may be the underlying mechanism. Since this altered sensitivity has been reported even in patients with normal renin hypertension, it is likely that patients with low-renin hypertension are not a distinct subset but rather form part of a continuum of patients with essential hypertension.

High-renin essential hypertension　Approximately 15 percent of patients with essential hypertension have plasma renin levels elevated above the normal range. It has been suggested that plasma renin plays an important role in the pathogenesis of the elevated blood pressure in these patients. However, most studies have documented that saralasin significantly reduces blood pressure in less than half of these patients. This has led some investigators to postulate that the elevated renin levels and blood pressure may both be secondary to an increased activity of the adrenergic system. It has been proposed that, in those patients with angiotensin-dependent high-renin hypertension whose arterial pressures are lowered by saralasin, the mechanism responsible for the increased renin and, therefore, the hypertension is a compensatory hyperreninemia secondary to a decreased adrenal responsiveness to angiotensin II.

3. Eeffects of Hypertension

For nearly 80 years it has been known that patients with hypertension die prematurely. The most common cause of death is heart disease, with strokes and renal failure also frequently occurring, particularly in those with significant retinopathy.

1) Effects on Heart: Cardiac compensation for the excessive work load imposed by increased systemic pressure is at first sustained by left ventricular hypertrophy. Ultimately, the function of this chamber deteriorates, it dilates, and the symptoms and signs of heart failure appear. Angina pectoris may also occur because of accelerated coronary arterial disease and/or increased myocardial oxygen requirements as a consequence of the increased myocardial mass, which exceeds the capacity of the coronary circulation. On physical examination the heart is enlarged and has a prominent left ventricular impulse. The sound of aortic closure is accentuated, and there may be a faint murmur of aortic regurgitation. Presystolic (atrial, fourth) heart

10

sounds appear frequently in hypertensive heart disease, and a protodiastolic (ventricular, third heart) sound or summation gallop rhythm may be present. Electrocardiographic changes of left ventricular hypertrophy are common; evidence of ischemia or infarction may be observed late in the disease. The majority of deaths due to hypertension result from myocardial infarction or congestive heart failure.

2) Neurologic Effects: The neurologic effects of long-standing hypertension may be divided into retinal and central nervous system changes. Because the retina is the only tissue in which the arteries and arterioles can be examined directly, repeated ophthalmoscopic examination provides the opportunity to observe the progress of the vascular effects of hypertension. The Keith-Wagener-Barker classification of the retinal changes in hypertension has provided a simple and excellent means for serial evaluation of the hypertensive patient. Increasing severity of hypertension is associated with focal spasm and progressive general narrowing of the arterioles, as well as the appearance of hemorrhages, exudates, and papilledema. These retinal lesions often produce scotomata, blurred vision, and even blindness, especially in the presence of papilledema or hemor-

rhages of the macular area. Hypertensive lesions may develop acutely and, if therapy results in significant reduction of blood pressure, may show rapid resolution. Rarely, these lesions resolve without therapy. In contrast, retinal arteriolosclerosis results from endothelial and muscular proliferation, and it accurately reflects similar changes in other organs. Sclerotic changes do not develop as rapidly as hypertensive lesions, not do they regress appreciably with therapy. As a consequence of increased wall thickness and rigidity, sclerotic arterioles distort and compress the veins as they cross within their common fibrous sheath, and the reflected light streak from the arterioles is changed by the increased opacity of the vessel wall.

Central nervous system dysfunction also occurs frequently in patients with hypertension. Occipital headaches, most often in the morning, are among the most prominent early symptoms of hypertension. Dizziness, lightheadedness, vertigo, tinnitus, and dimmed vision or syncope may also be observed, but the more serious manifestations are due to vascular occlusion or hemorrhage.

3) Renal Effects: Arteriolosclerotic lesions of the afferent and efferent arteriloes and the golmerular capil-

lary tufts are the most common renal vascular lesions in hypertension and result in decreased glomerular filtration rate and tubular dysfunction proteinuria and microscopic hematuria occur because of glomerular lesions, and approximately 10 percent of the deaths secondary to hypertension result from renal failure. Blood loss in hypertension occurs not only from renal lesions, hemoptysis, and metrorrhagia also occurs most frequently in these patients.

4. Treatment

Virtually every patient with a diastolic arterial pressure exceeding 90 mmHg is a candidate for diagnostic studies and for subsequent treatment.

General measures(Table 1)　Nondrug therapeutic intervention is probably indicated in all patients with sustained hypertension and probably most with labile hypertension. the general measures employed include (1) relief of stress, (2) diet, (3) regular exercise, and (4) control of other risk factors contributing to the development of arteriosclerosis. Relief of emotional and environmental stress is one of the reasons for the improvement in hypertension that occurs when the patient is hospitalized. Though it is usually impossible to extricate the hypertensive patient from all internal and external stresses, he or she should be advised to avoid any unnecessary tensions. In rare instances it may be appropriate to recommend a change of job or of life-style. Recently it has been suggested that relaxation techniques may also lower arterial pressure. However, it is uncertain that these techniques alone have much long-term effect. Dietary management has three aspects:

1) Because of the documented efficacy of sodium restriction and volume contraction in lowering blood pressure, patients previously were instructed to curtail sodiun intake drastically. The advent of effective oral diuretics provided an additional method of decreasing body sodium stores and led some to suggest that sodium restriction was no longer necessary.

However, a number of reports have documented that while mild sodium restriction has little, if any, direct action on blood pressure, it significantly potentiates the effectiveness of nearly all antihypertensive agents. Thus, the most practical approach now is to advise mild dietary sodium restriction (up to 5 g NaCl per day).

Table 1　Treatment of patients with hypertension

GENERAL MEASURES

---

1 Relief of stress (relaxation techniques)

2 Dietary control

　a Restrict sodium chloride to 4 - 6 g per day

　b Restrict calories

　c Restrict cholesterol and sturated fats

3 Regular isotonic exercise

4 Stop cigarette smoking

DRUG THERAPY

Step 1: Thiazide diuretic

Step 2: Add an antiadrenergic agent: blocker, methyldopa, or reserpine

Step 3: Add a vasodilator: hydralazine or captopril

Step 4: Add guanethidine or substitute clonidine or prazosin for a step 2 drug

---

2) Caloric restriction should be urged for the patient who is overweight. Some obese patients will show a significant reduction in pressure simply as a consequence of weight loss.

3) A moderate restriction in intake of cholesterol and saturated fats is recommended on the suggestive evidence that such a diet may diminish the incidence of arteriosclerotic somplicationc. Regular exercise is indicated within the limits of the patient's cardiovascular

status. Not only is exercise helpful in controlling weight, but in addition there is evidence that physical conditioning itself may lower arterial pressure. Isotonic exercises (jogging, swimming) are better than isometric exercises (weight lifting) since, if anything, the latter raises arterial pressure. The dietary managemant outlined above is aimed at the control of other risk factors. Probably the most significant additional step that could be taken in this area would be to covince the smoker to give up cigarettes.

Drug therapy (Table 2)　To make rational use of antihypertensive drugs, the sites and mechanisms of their action must be understood. In general, there are four classes or drugs: diuretics, antiadrenergic agents, vasodilators, and angiotensin blockers.

1) Diurenics　Drugs active on the renal tubules affect arterial pressure primarily by causing sodium diuresis and volume depletion. The thiazides are the most frequently used and most extensively investigated members of this group, and their early effect certainly is related to the diuresis. A reduction in peripheral vascular resistance also has been reported by some workers to be important in the long term. Thiazide diuretics form the cornerstone of most therapeutic programs designed to

16

lower arterial pressure and are usually effective within 3 to 4 days . Their most frequent side effects are hypokalemia due to renal potassium loss, hyperuricemia due to uric acid retention, and carbohydrate intolerance. The more potent diuretics, furosemide and ethacrynic acid, also have been shown to be antihypertensive but have been less extensively used for this purpose primarily because of their shorter duration of acrion. Spironolactone causes renal sodium loss by blocking the effect of endogenous mineralocorticoids, and therefore it may be more effective in patients whose mineralocorticoids are present in excess, e. g. ,primary or secondary aldosteronism. Although they do not compete directly with aldosterone, triamterene and amiloride act at the same site as spirononlactone to impede sodium reabsorption and are effective in the same situations as spironolactone. Any of these three potassium-sparing diuretics can also be given along with thiazide diuretics to minimize renal potassium loss.

(2) Antiadrenergic agents These drugs act at one or more sites either centrally on the vasomotor center, in peripheral neurons modifying catecholamine release, or by blocking adrenergic receptor sites on target tissues that appear to have predominant central actions

are clonidine and methyldopa. These drugs and their metabolites are predominantly alpha-receptor agonists. Stimulation of alpha receptors in the vasomotor centers of the brain reduces sympathetic outflow, thereby reducing arterial pressure. Usually a fall in cardiac output and heart rate also occurs, more commonly with clonidine, but the baroreceptor reflex is intact. Thus, postural symptoms are absent. However, rebound hypertension may rarely occur when these drugs, particularly clonidine, are stopped. This is probably secondary to the increase in norepinephrine release which had been inhibited by these agents secondary to their agonist effect on presynaptic alpha receptors.

Another class of antiadrenergic agents is the ganglionic blocking drugs. These compounds block ganglionic transmission in the autonomic nervous system. They have little effect when the patient is supine, but they prevent reflex vasoconstriction in the upright position. Ganglionic blocking agents interfere with parasympathetic as well as sympathetic function, and this results in such side effects as impairment of visual accommodation, paralytic ileus, retention of urine, and failure of erection and ejaculation. Because of these problems, ganglionic blocking agents are now usually

18

reserved for the rapid lowering of arterial pressure by parenteral administration of the short-acting agent trimethaphan in patients with severe hypertension.

Various drugs act at postganglionic nerve endings. The rauwolfia alkaloids are the oldest members of the group, their long-term effect results from their ability to inhibit the storage of norepinephrine within the vesicles in adrenergic nerve endings, thus leading to depletion of catecholamine stores. When given parenterally, they also have a direct effect on vascular smooth muscle. The rauwolfia alkaloids, like the other drugs of this class, exhibit the side effects that result from the unopposed activity of the parasympathetic nervous system, including nasal congestion, diarrhea, impairment of sexual function, and increased gastric secretion. Depression is the most serious side effect of the rauwolfia alkaloids; this is most likely to occur in elderly patients. The rauwolfia alkaloids are most helpful in treatment by the oral route of mild to moderate hypertension. Guanethidine blocks the release of norepinephrine from the sympathetic nerve endings. It has a greater postural effect than the other drugs that work at the nerve endings, and orthostatic hypotension is a frequent side effect. However, centrally mediated side effects (sedation, depression)are infrequently observed since guanethidine has a low lipid solubility and therefore, only poorly enters the central nervous system.

The last group of drugs affecting the adrenergic system are those which block the peripheral adrenergic receptors, either alpha or beta. Phentolamine and phenoxybenzamine block the action of norepinephrine at alpha-adrenergic receptor sites. While the above two compounds block both pre-and postsynaptic alpha receptors, the former action accounts for the tolerance which develops. Thus, presynaptic alpha action remains, suppressing norepinephrine release.

A variety of effective beta-adrenergic receptor blocking agents are available which block sympathetic effects on the heart and should be most effective in reducing cardiac output and in lowering arterial pressure when there is increased cardiac sympathetic nerve activity. In addition, they block the adrenergic nerve-mediated release of renin from the renal juxtaglomerular cells, and this action may be an important component of their blood pressure-lowering action. Beta-adrenergic blockers are particularly useful when employed in conjunction with vascular smooth-muscle relaxants, tend to evoke a reflex increase in myocardial contractility, and with diuretics, the administration of which often results in an elevation of circulating renin activity. In practice, beta blockers appear to be effective even when there is no evidence of increased sympathetic tone with about one-half or more of all patients showing a fall in pressure. However, these agents can precipitate congestive heart failure and asthma in susceptible.

Table 2 Drugs used in treatment of hypertension-listed according to site of action

Site of action	Drug	Dosage	Indications
DIURETICS			
Renal tubule	Thiazides	Depends on specific drug	Mild hypertension, as adjunct in treatment
	Hydrochloro—thiazide	Oral: 25-50 mg daily or twice daily	of moderate to severe hypertension
	Furosemide	Oral: 20-40 mg daily or twice daily	Mild hypertension, as adjunct in severe or malignant hypertension

	Ethacrynic acid	Oral: 25-50 mg twice dialy	Mild hypertension, as adjunct in severe or malignant hypertension
	Spironolactone	Oral: 25-100mg three or four times daily	Hypertension due to hypermineralo-corticoidism, adjunct to thiazi detherapy
	Triamterene	Oral: 100mg one to three times daily	Hypertension due to hypermineralo-corticoidism, adjunct to thiazide therapy

ANTIADRENERGIC AGENTS

Central	Clonidine	Oral: 0. 1-0. 6mg two to four times daily	Mild to moderate hypertension, renal disease with hypertension
	Methyldopa (also acts by blocking sympathetic nerves)	Oral: 250-750 mg three or four times daily IV: 250-1000 mg every 4-6 h (tolerance may develop)	Mild to moderate hypertension (oral), malignat hypertension(IV)
	Secatives and tranquilizers		Tense or anxious patient with hypertension
	Diazepam	Oral: 2-10mg four times daily	

Site of action	Drug	Dosage	Indications
Autonomic gangina	Trimethaphan	IV: 1-10 mg/min	Severe or malignant hypertension
Nerve endings	Rauwolfia alka loids		Mild to moderate hypertension in young patient
	Reserpinr	Oral:0.1-0.5 mg daily	
	Guanethidine	Oral:10-300 mg daily	Moderate to severe hypertension
Alpha receptors	Phentolamine	IV: 1-5 mg	Suspected or proved pheochromocytoma
	Phenoxy— benzamine	Oral:10-50 mg once or twice daily (tolerance may develop)	Proved pheo- chromocytoma
Beta receptors	Propranolol	Oral:10-120mg two to four times daily	Mild to moderte Moder the hypertension (especially with evidence for hyperdynamic circulation),adjunct to hydralazine therapy
	Metoprolol	Oral:50-225 mg twice daily	

VASODILATORS

			As adjunct in
Vascular smooth muscle	Hydralazine	Oral: 10-75 mg four times daily IV or IM: 10-50 mg every 6 h (tolerance may develop)	treatment ot moderate to severe hypertension (oral), malignant hypertension (IV or IM), renal disease with hypertension
	Nitroprusside	IV: 0. 5-8 (kg/kg)/min	Malignant hypertension

-CONVERTING ENZYME INHIBITOR

	Captopril	Oral: 10-150 mg three times daily	Treatment-resistant hypertension: renal artery stenosis

Individuals and must be used with caution in diabetics receiving hypoglycemic therapy because they inhibit the usual sympathetic responses to hypoglycemia. Cardios-elective beta-blocking agents (so-called beta$_1$ blockers) have been developed (metoprolol, atenolol)which may be superior to nonselective beta blockers such as propranolol in patients with bronchospasm.

(3) Vasodilators: Hydralzine is the most versatile of the drugs that cause direct relaxation of vascular

smooth muscle, it is effective both orally and parenterally, acting mainly on arterial resistance, rather than on venous capacitance vessels, as evidenced by lack of postural changes. Unfortunately, the effect of hydralazine on peripheral resistance is partly negated by reflex increases in sympathetic discharges that raise heart rate and cardiac output. These limit the usefulness of hydralazine, especialy in patients with severe coronary artery disease. However, the efficacy of hydralazine can be increased if it is given in conjunction with beta blockers or drugs such as methyldopa, clonidine, or reserpine, all of which blockr efoex sympathetic stimulation of the heart. A serious side effect of doses of hydralazine exceeding 300 mg per day has been the production of a lupus erythmatosus-like syndrome.

Nitroprusside given intravenously also acts as a direct vasodilator, with onset and offset of actions that are almost immediate. these latter two drugs are useful only for the treatment of hypertensive emergencies.

(4) Angiotensin blockers　Drugs from several of the categories discussed above have been shown to possess an additional action resulting in inhibition of renin secretion. These include clonidine, reserpine, methyldopa, and propranolol, with clonidine and propranolol

25

being the most effective. There is also a group of analogues of angiotensin II, e. g. , saralasin, that act by antagonizing the effects of angiotensin II; these polypeptides require parenteral administration and are not useful for chronic management. A third group of drugs in this class are those which inhibit the enzyme converting angiotensin I into angiotensin II, e. g, captopril. Data on these converting-enzyme inhibitors are still limited. However, these agents are extremely promising because they not only inhibit the generation of a potent vasoconstrictor (agniotensin II) but also retard the degradation of a potent vasodilator (bradykinin) and may alter prostaglandin production. They are especially useful in renal or renovascular hypertension, as well as in accelerated and malignant hypertension. Their value in milder, uncomplicated hypertension will depend on the incidence and severity of adverse effects with prolonged use.

Section 2
Malignant hypertension

In addition to marked blood pressure elevation in association with papilledema and retinal hemorrhages and exudates, the full-blown picture of malignant hypertension may include manifestations of hypertensive encephalopathy, such as severe headache, vomiting, visual disturbances (including transient blindness), transient paralyses, convulsions, stupor, and coma. These have been attributed to spasms of cerebral vessels and to cerebral edema. In some patients who have died, multiple small thrombi have been found in the cerebral vessels. Cardiac decompensation and rapidly declining renal function are other critical features of malignant hypertension. Oliguria may, in fact, be the presenting feature. The vascular lesion characteristic of malignant hypertension in fibrinoid necrosis of the walls of small ateries and arterioles, and this can be reversed by effective antihypertensive therapy.

The pathogenesis of malignant hypertension is unknown. However, at least two independent processes, dilatation of cerebral arteries and generalized arteriolar fibrinoid necrosis, contribute to the associated signs and symptoms.

About 1 percent of hypertensive patients develop the malignant phase, which occurs in the course of both essential and secondary hypertension. Rarely it is the first recognized manifestaion of the blood pressure problem. The average age at diagnosis is 40, and men are more often affected than women. Prior to the availability of effective therapy, life expectancy after diagnosis of malignant hypertension was less than 2 years, with most deaths being due to renal failure, cerebral hemorrhage or congestive heart failure. With the advent of effective antihypertensive therapy, at least half of patients survive for more than 5 years.

Malignant hypertension is a medical emergency and requires immediate therapy. The initial aim of therapy should be to reduce diastolic pressure toward, but not below, 90 mmHg. The drugs available for treatment of malignant hypertension can be divided into two groups on the basis of time of onset of action (Table 3). Those in the first group act within a few minutes but are not satisfactory for long-term management. If the patient is having convulsions, if arterial pressure must be reduced rapidly, then one from the immediate-acting group should be used. Diazoxide is the easiest to administer, for no individual titration of dosage is required. A dose of 300 mg is given rapidly intravenously, and the antihypertensive effect is noted in 1 to 2 min. The same dose can be repeated when the pressure begins to rise, usually after several hours. In an occasional patient, pressure may drop below normal levels after diazoxide administration. Because of this, some physicians use a modified program, giving 150 mg rather than 300 mg initially, followed by a second 150mg dose in 5 min if the blood pressure response has been minimal. It should not be used in patients who may have a dissecting aneurysm. The other two agents in this group require continuous infusion and close monitoring. Nitroprusside is given by continuous intravenous infusion at a dose of 0.5 to 8.0 (μg/kg) min. It has the advantage over the ganglionic blockers of not being associated with the development of tachyphylaxis and can be utilized for days with few side effects. The dosage must be controlled with an infusion pump. Trimethaphan, a ganglionic blocker, is given at a rate of 1 to 15 mg/min. The patient should be in the sitting position, and the pressure should be monitored closely preferably in an intensive care unit.

Patients given any of these agents should also receive other medications effective for long-term control. Those in the second group require 30 min or more to obtain full effect, but have the advantage of being satisfactory for subsequent oral administration and for long-term management of the patient's hypertension (Table 3). If such a delay in attainment of full effect is acceptable intravenous methyldopa is an effective drug with which to begin therapy if symptoms of encephalopathy are absent. A dose of 500mg in 100 to 200 ml 5% dextrose in water is given intravenously over 30 min; if the effect is inadequate in 2 to 4 h, a second dose of 500 to 1000mg is given. Additional intravenous doses may then be given every 6 h until the pressure is stabilized. Intravenous hydralazine is effective in many patients within 10 min; an effective protocol involves giving 10-mg doses intravenously every 10 to 15 min until the desired effect has been obtained or until a total of 50 mg has been administered. The total required for response may then be repeated intramuscularly or intravenously every 6 h. Hydralazine should be used with caution in patients with significant coronary artery disease and should be avoided in patients evidencing myocardial ischemia or dissecting aneurysm.

The converting-enzyme inhibitor, captopril, while promising in preliminary studies is still under investigation.

The potent diuretics furosemide and ethacrynic acid are important adjuncts to the therapy just discussed. Given either orally or intravenously, they serve to maintain sodium diuresis in the face of a falling arterial pressure, and thus will speed recovery from enciphalopathy and congestive heart failure as well as maintain sensitivity to the primary antihypertensive drug. Digitalis also is indicated if there is evidence of cardiac decompensation.

In patients with malignant hypertension in whom the existence of pheochromocytoma is suspected, urine should be collected for measurement of the products of catecholamine metabolism and drugs which might release additional catecholamines, such as methyldopa, reserpine, and guanethidine, must be avoided. The parenteral drug of choice in these patients is phentolamine administered with care to avoid a precipitous reduction in arterial pressure.

Table 3 Therapeutic agents used to treat malignant hypertension

Drug	Route	Onset	Peak	Duration
		Time course of action		
IMMEDIATE ONSET				
Diazoxide	IV bluus	1-3min	2-4min	4-12h
Nitroprusside	Continuous IV	<1min	1-2min	2-5min
Trimethaphan	Continuous IV	<1min	1-2min	2-5min
DEIAYED ONSET				
Hydralazine	IV, IM	10-20min	20-40min	2-6h
Methyidopa	IV	1-3h	3-5h	2-12h
Reserpine	IM	2-3h	3-4h	6-24h

In general, traditional Chinese treatment of hypertension lowers the blood pressure less but relieves hypertensive symptoms better than Western medicine. Therefore, combined TCM and Western medicine is a logical-approach for hypertension.

Chapter Two

DIFFERENTIATION AND
TREATMENT OF COMMON SYNDROMES

Hypertension is included in the categories of "xuan yun"(vertigo)and "tou tong"(headache). It is common thought that hypertension occurs when incoordination between yin and yang is caused by impairment of seven modes of emotion ,improper diet, internal damage and deficiency. The main injured visera are heart, liver and kidney.

Section 1
Main points of pathogenesis

1. Sthenia of liver yang

It is usually postulated that long-term emotional upsets or grief easily lead to stagnation of the liver-energy with formation of evil fire, mainfested as headache, dizziness, tinnitus, restlessness, flushed face and others. Overexertion or body debility and general hypofunction may induce consumption of blood or deficiency of yin and gradually lead to the inequality of yin and yang in which the yin is unable to inhibit yang-energy and over-activity of yang ensues, and in turn, the hyperactivity of yang may further consumes the yin-fluid which further results in development of liver yang hyperactivity due to deficiency of yin-fluid. Sthenia of liver-yang usually occurs in mild hypertension.

2. The deficiency of the liver-yin and kidney-yin

Liver and kidney is said to come from the same origin. Between them there are the mutual supply of nutrients and the close relationship. Liver stores blood and kidney stores essence. The blood and essence are able to transform each other. In sufficiency of kidney-yin usually insufficiency of liver-yin and vice versa, which would lead to the deficiency of the liver-yin and kidney-yin, It usually presents in some of patients with hypertension and probably accounts for the hypertension in these patients.

3. Deficiency of yin leading to hyperactivity of yang

It is a morbid condition due to the consumption of essence, blood and body fluid, which can lead to the inequality of yin and yang, in which the yin is unable to inhibit yang-energy and over-activity of yang ensues, and, in turn, the hyperactivity of yang may further consumes the yin-fluid. In clinic, the diagnosis may be established by concomitant appearance of the deficiency of liver-yin and kidney-yin accompanying with sthenia of liver-yang.

4. Deficiency of heart-yin

Heart-yin is the nutritious fluid of the heart and a component of blood. It has a close relation to the heart-blood physiologically and pathologically, and also to the condition of lung-yin and kidney-yin. deficiency of kidney-yin may cause that water fails to inhibit fire which will gradually lead to an excess of fire and eventually result in the deficiency of heart-yin. The common features, such as palpitation, insomnia, dreaminess and amnesia, are sought in the most of patients with hypertension.

5. Deficiency of both yin and yang

It is a morbid condition characterized by simultaneously occurrence of deficiency of yin and yang and usually seen in the later stage of hypertension. The occurrence results from prolonged hypertension with improper treatment. The causes are that yang is involved by deficient yin such as kidney damage resulting in chronic renal failure. This type is less than another types in hypertensive patients.

6. Deficiency of both vital energy and yin: It is a morbid condition of damage of both yin fluid and yang-energy occurring in the course of hypertension in moderate depth. Vital energy is the functions of various organs and tissues of the body, which is in cluded in the categories of yang in Chinese traditional medicine. Deficiency of vital energy may cause hypofunction of viscera and lowering of metabolism due to insufficiency of yang-energy with failure to warm and nourish the viscera, manifesting as pale complexion, dizziness, tinnitus, palpitation, shortness of breath, lassitude and spontaneous sweating. Deficiency of yin may cause hyperactivity of fire, manifesting as hot feeling of the palms and soles, red lips, dry mouth, oliguria with yellowish urine, constipation, red and uncoated tongue, headache and others. In an individual patient when there are simultaneously symptoms of both dificiency of vital energy and deficiency of yin, the diagnosis of this type may be established by carefully examination.

36

7. Maladjustment of chong and ren channels

It may result from impairment of the liver and kidney, elderly and climacteric irregular menstruation and is usually seen in the female patients with hypertension. Irregular menstruation usually occurs preceding t0 the amenorrhea. In the menstrual period, there are obviously fluctuation of the blood pressure and general malaise, which easily induce to elevate the level of the blood pressure.

Section 2

Differentiation and treatment of common syndromes

1. Sthenia of liver-yang

Main symptoms and signs: Dizziness, headache, head distension, vexation temperamental tendency, flushed eyes, bitter taste, red tongue with yellow fur, taut and forceful pulse.

Therapeutic principle: Calming the liver and subduing hyperactivity of liver-yang

Recipe: Modified Decoction of Gastrodia and Uncaria.

Interpretation: Gastrodia tuber, Uncaria stem with hooks and abalone shell calm the liver to stop the wind as principal drugs. Capejasmine fruit and scutellaria root clear away heat and purge fire from the liver channel as assistant drugs. Motherwort promotes blood circulation and induces diuresis. A chyranthes root ensures proper down ward flow of the blood from the head. Bark of eucommia, loranthus mulberry mistletoe nourish the liver and kidney. Fleece-flower stem and poria with host wood tranquilize the mind.

2. Deficiency of the liver-yin and kidney-yin

Main symptoms and signs: Headache, vertigo, tinnitus, dryness of eyes, vexation, palpitation, insomnia, poor memory, feverish sensation in the palms and soles, aching and lassitude of the loins and legs, dry mouth, red tongue with a little or no fur, fine and string-like pulse.

Theraprutic principle: Nourishing yin and suppressing hyperactive yang.

Recipe: Modified Decoction of Fleece-Flower for Longerity.

Ingredients: fleece-flower root (Radix Polygoni Multiflori) 15g, dry rehmannia root (Radix Rehmanniae) 12g, wolfberry fruit (Fructus Lycii) 12g, tortoise-Plastronglue (Golla Plastri Testudinis) 15g, eucommi bark (Cortex Eucommiae) 9g, loranthus mulberry mistletoe (Ramulus Loranthi) 15g, Xhyenrhwa root (Achyranthis Bidentatae) 15g, magnetite (magnetitum) 15 — 30g, Parched wild jujuba seed (Semen ziziphi Sprinosae) 12g, chryanthemum flower (Flos Chrysanthemi) 9g.

3. Deficiency of yin leading to hyperactivity of yang

Main symptoms and signs consist of both deficiency of liver and kidney and hyperactivity of liver-yang.

Therapeutic principle: Nourishing yin and suppressing sthenic yang.

Recipe: Decoction of Wolfberry-Chrysanthemum-Rehmannia.

Interpretation: Decoction of wolfberry-chrysanthemum-Rehmannia Consists of Decoction of six drugs Including Rehmannia combined with wolfberry fruit and chrysanthemum flower, 9 grams respectively, which have function of nourishing yin and calming the liver.

4. Deficiency of heart-yin

It is usually combined with deficiency of kidney-yin. The main symptoms and signs are composed of vexation, palpitation, mental weariness, nocturnal emission, amnesia, dry stools, orolingual boil, reddened tongue with little fur, thready and rapid pulse.

Therapeutic principle: Nourishing kidney and tonifying heart.

Recipe: Modified cardiotonic pill.

Interpretation: Dried rehmannia root is used in large dosage to nourish yin and blood, tonify the kidney and the heart; combined with Figwort root as principal drugs to nourishe yin and clear pathogenic fire to get the deficiency-fire suppressed and mind tranquilized. Red sage root, Chinese angelica root, Ginseng and Tuckahoe invigorate qi, enrich the blood and tranquilize the mind. Arborvitae seed, wild or spiny jujuba seed and polygala root reinforce the heart and the spleen to tranquilize the mind. Lucid asparagus and lilyturf root, sweet in taste and cold in nature, produce an moistening effect to clear deficiency-fire. Magnolia vine fruit astringes qi and promotes the production of the body fluid to avoid the dissipation of the heart-qi. Root of balloonflower carries all the ingredients in the recipe upward. Cinnabar tranquilizes the mind. The joint use of all the drugs in the recipe can get yin and blood enriched, the five of deficiency type reduced, thus, with the mind tranquilized spontaneously.

5. Deficiency of both yin and yang

Main symptoms and signs: Dizziness, tinnitus, amnesia, palpitation, lassitude, soreness of the loins and knees. Inclination to yang deficiency gives rise to cold extremities, pale tongue and deep thready pulse, while inclination to yin deficiency brings about dysphoria with feverish sensation in the chest, palms and soles, red tongue and fine rapid pulse.

Therapeutic Principle: Nourishing yin and restoring yang.

Recipe: (Modified Decoction of Curculigo and Epimedium)

Modified Bolus for Tonifying the Kidney-qi.

Interpretation: Dried rehmannia root, Chinese yam and Dogwood fruit are all used as tonics, the first replenishing the kidney-yin while the second and the third nourishing the liver and spleen to reinforce the effect of the first one. Oriental water plantain and poria play their part in removing dampness and promoting diuresis. Moutan bark has the effect of removing liver-fire and is coordinated with the invigorators for kidney-yang to produce the consequence of coexistance of both invigorating and purging action for the purpose of getting rid of the greasy side involved in the invigorating action.

6. Deficiency of both vital energy and yin

Main symptoms and signs: Lassitude due to deficiency of qi, disinclination to talk, intolerance of cold, poor appetite, loose stool, or puffy face and edema of limbs, pale and tender tongue and deep, thready and weak pulse.

Therapeutic principle: Replenishing qi, nourishing yin and strengthening the spleen and removing dampness.

Recipe: Modified prescriptions of Docoction of Four Noble Drugs and powder of Five drugs with Poria.

Intepretation: Decoction of Four Noble Drugs has four ingredients in the recipe. Ginseng possesses the effect of invigorating primordial qi and acts as a principal drug. Bighead atractylodes rhizome is effective for strengthening the spleen and eliminating dampness. Poria exerts the part of an adjuvant drug in achieving the effect of strengthening the spleen. Prepared licorice root is used as a guiding drug for regulating the middle-warmer.

Powder of Five Drugs with Poria is used as removing dampness by promoting diuresis. Poria and polyporus umbellatus strengthen the effect of removing excessive fluid. Bighead atractylodes rhizome enriches the spleen to transport and transform warm and dampness, both being used as assistant drugs. Cassia twig can relieve the exterior syndrome by dispelling pathogenic cold and warm yang to expel qi, acting as an adjuvant drug.

7. Maladjustment of chong and ren channels

Before or during menstruation, before or after menopause, women may have some symptoms including headache, dizziness, restlessness, insomnia, distension in sternocostal region, general malaise and fluctuation of blood pressure, taut and thready pulse.

Therapeutic principle: Regulate the chong and ren channels.

Recipe: Modified Ease Powder.

Interpretation: Bupleurum root soothes the liver to disperse the depressed qi. Chinese angelica root and white peony root nourish the blood and the liver. The joint use of the three drugs is able to treat the primary cause of stagnation of the liver-qi and deficiency of the blood. Tuckahole and Bighead atractylodes rhizome strengthen the middle-warmer and reinforce the spleen so as to enrich the source of growth and development of the qi and blood. Roasted ginger regulates the stomach and warms the middle-warmer. Peppermint assists Bupleurum root in soothing the liver to disperse the depressed qi, prepared licorice root can coordinate the effects of all the drugs in the recipe.

Section 3

Clinical Case Reports

CASE 1

Abnormal Rising of Liver-heat

Qiu, a 52-year-old male, came to the hospital on account of dizziness and headache in the preceding more than 3 years.

The patient had been diagnosed hypertension by another hospital. The blood pressure was 24. 8/14. 9kPa(186/112mmHg). Verticilum, Reserpinum, etc. failed to take favorable effects. The condition developed in the last a few days because of emotional stress. He felt dizziness and distending pain in the head, dry mouth and bitter taste, and occasional feeling of heat rising to the top of the head. On examination, the patient was a well- nourished male with fat build. The complexion was red. Yellow and greasy fur, strong, smooth and taut pulse.

The patient was diagnosed vertigo caused by stagnated liver-energy changing into fire which interrupted the vital energy circulation of the head.

Therapeutic principle of clearing away the liver-fire was performed.

Recipe:

gentian root, Radix Gentianae 12g

cape jasmine fruit, Fructus Gardeniae 15g

scutellaria root, Radix Scutellariae 15g

dried rehmannia root, Radix Rehmanniae 15g

oriental waterplantain rhizome, Rhizoma Alismatis 15g

hooked uncaria, Ramulus Uncariae cum Uncis 15g

loranthus mulberry mistletoe, Ramulus Loranthi 15g

chrysanthemum flower, Flos Chrysanthemi 20g

prunella spike, Spica Prunellae 30g

fleece-flower stem, Caulis Polygoni Multiflori 30g

After taking two doses of the above recipe, the

headache and dizziness were alleviated in a considerable degree, and the other symptoms were relieved at the same time. The blood pressure was lowered to 20. 3/ 13. 1kPa (152/98mmHg). He was able to go to work two months later.

Explanation: The symptoms and signs of dizziness, distending pain in the head, red complexion, dry mouth and bitter taste, red tongue with yellow and greasy fur were caused by the abnormal rising of liver-fire. Radix Gentianae, Capejasmine, Radix Scutellariae, Spica Prunellae can clear away the liver-fire; Flos Chrysanthemi, Ramulus Uncariae cum Uncis lower the abnormal rising of liver-heat; Rhizoma Alismatis can clear away heat through urination; Caulis Polygoni Multiflori can calm the mind; Radix Rehmanniae and Ramulus Loranthi invigorate the kidney-yin.

CASE 2

Abnormal Rising of Liver- fire Combined with Damp-heat Stagnated in the Liver and Gallbladder

Li, a 34-year-old male, came to the hospital because of dizziness and headache that began one month earlier.

46

The patient was well until one month previously, when he began to suffer from dizziness and headache, accompanied with palpitation, dreaminess, irritability, aversion to light, yellow urine, etc.. The symptoms increased in recent days. On examination, the tongue was red with yellow and greasy fur, slippery and taut pulse. The blood pressure was 26. 7/19. 7kPa (200/148mmHg). The urinary protein was $+++$ positive; NPN 60mg; funduscopy revealed papilledema. A diagnosis of accelerated hypertension was made by another hospital. Some kind of drugs were then used, however, with no effect taken.

A diagnosis of headache and dizziness due to abnormal rising of liver-fire and damp- heat in the liver and gallbladder was made.

Therapeutic principles of clearing away the liver-fire and resolving damp-heat from the liver and gallbladder were performed.

Recipe:

gentian root, Radix Gentianae 12g

cape jasmine fruit, Fructus Gardeniae 12g

scutellaria root, Radix Scutellariae 15g

thorowax root, Radix Bupleuri 12g

grassleaf sweetflag rhizome, Rhizoma Acori

Graminei 12g

    prunella spike, Spica Prunellae 30g

    dragon's bone, Os Draconis Fossilia Ossis Mastodi
24g

    oyster shell, Concha Ostreae 24g

    batryticated silkworm, Bombyx Batryticatus 15g

    plantain seed, Semen Plantaginis 10g

    liquorice root, Radix Glycyrrhizae 6g

    oriental waterplantain rhizome, Rhizoma Alismatis 10g

After taking two doses of the above recipe, the patient felt the symptoms greatly alleviated. The blood pressure was 17. 3/12. 0kPa (130/90mmHg) . The quantity of Os Draconis Fossilia Ossis Mastodi and Concha Ostreae increased to 30g each and after taking another two doses the symptoms were relieved and the blood pressure was lowered to 16. 0/11. 5kPa (120/86mmHg). No relapse was claimed at a follow- up two months later. Examination revealed normal blood pressure, negative result of urinary protein, and NPN 35mg. Funduscopy revealed no papilledema.

    Explanation: Fructus gardeniae, Radix Gentianae, Radix Scutellariae and Spica Prunellae can clear away liver-fire; Semen Plantaginis and Rhizoma Alismatis can resolve damp and heat; Bombyx Batry ticatus and Rhizoma Acori Graminei remove phlegm in order to prevent the complication of hypertensive cerebral disorders.

CASE 3

Abnormal Rising of Liver- fire Combined with Sthenia-syndrome of Stomach

Gan, a 48-year-old female, came to the hospital on account of hypertension that began 5 years earlier.

The patient was well until 5 years previously, when she began to suffer from hypertension marked by dull pain in the head, dry mouth with bitter taste, saburra, insomnia and dreaminess, distending pain in the abdomen, and constipation.

On examination, the paitient was a well- nourished woman of strong build. The blood pressure was 24. 0/14. 1kPa(180/106mmHg). Thick yellow tongue fur, taut and strong pulse.

A TCM diagnosis of headache due to abnormal rising of liver-fire and sthenia of stomach was made.

Therapeutic principles of clearing away liver-fire and relaxing the bowels were performed.

Recipe:

rough gentian, Radix Gentianae 10g

dried root of rehmannia, Radix Rehmanniae 10g

chrysanthemum, Flos Chrysanthemi 10g

shell of abalone, Concha Haliotidis 10g

skullcap root,.Radix Scutellariae 12g

cape jasmine fruit, Fructus Gardeniae 12g

Asiatic plantain seed, Semen Plantaginis 12g

fiveleaf akebia (stem), Caulis Akebiae 6g

henon bamboo leaf, Herba Lophatheri 6g

Chinaberry fruit, Fructus Meliae Toosendan 9g

licorice root, Radix Glycyrrhizae 3g

After taking three doses of the above recipe, all the symptoms were alleviated. The next day the patient complained of increased headache accompanied by irritability and distending pain in the abdomen, and constipation for 3 days. Rhubarb root (Radix et Rhizoma Rhei) 6g and mirabilite (Mirabilitum) 6g were added to the former recipe. After taking the other two doses the symptoms were alleviated in a considerable degree and the tongue fur recovered to normal. The blood pressure decreased to 18. 7/12. 0kPa (140/90mmHg).

CASE 4

Abnormal Rising of both Liver-yang and Liver-fire Combined with Phlegm-evil

Liu, a 70-year-old male, came to the hospital on April 2, 1983 on account of headache and dizziness which increased in the preceding two days.

The patient had been suffered from headache for many years. The condition developed two days before after he had had a quarrel over something which led to irritability and insomnia. The next morning he suffered severe headache and dizziness which forced him to stay in bed. The patient also complained of numbness of the left hand, dry mouth, numbness of the tongue tip, constipation and oliguria.

On examination, the patient revealed grey tongue fur, taut, slippery and rapid pulse. The blood pressure was 29.3/17.3kPa(220/130mmHg).

Differentiation: The condition was caused by abnormal rising of both liver-yang and liver-fire accompanied with phlegm-heat in the meridians and channels of organs. Cerebrovascular accident should be prevented.

Therapeutic principles of calming the liver, suppressing the yang hyperactivity, clearing away liver-fire, and resolving phlegm-heat were performed.

Recipe:

rough gentian, Radix Gentianae 10g

cape jasmine fruit, Fructus Gardeniae 10g

skullcap root, Radix Scutellariae 10g

oriental water plantain rhizome, Rhizoma Alismatis 10g

tabasheer, Concretio Silicea Bambusae 10g

rhubarb root, Radix et Rhizoma Rhei 10g

gambirplant, Ramulus Uncariae cum Uncis 10g

dried root of rehmannia, Radix Rehmanniae 20g

shell of abalone, Concha Haliotidis 20g

fossil fragments, Os Draconis 20g

oyster shell, Concha Ostreae 20g

After taking three doses of the above recipe, the symptoms and signs improved in a considerable degree. The constipation was removed and the urination recovered to normal. The numbness of the left hand and tongue tip disappeared. The patient got a good sleep and the dizziness was relieved. The tongue fur was yellowish and the pulse was slow and taut. The blood pressure was 24.0/13.3kPa(180/100mmHg). After taking over 20 doses of the recipe, all the symptoms were relieved and the blood pressure recovered to normal. No relapse was claimed at follow-ups.

CASE 5

Hyperactivity of Liver- yang and Asthenia of Kidney-yin

A 52-year-old male, came to the hospital on April 16, 1982 on account of increased headache that began 3 days earlier.

The patient was well until 3 days previously, when he suffered from the onset of increased distending pain in the head and severe dizziness, accompanied with soreness of the waist, fatigue in the knees, irritability, dry throat with a bitter taste, insomnia and dreaminess, oliguria, dry stools.

On examination, the tongue was dark red with thin yellow fur; the pulse was taut and rapid. The blood pressure was 26. 7/16. 0kPa(200/120mmHg). Fluoroscopy revealed left ventricular hypertrophy and projection of aortic arch.

The patient was diagnosed hypertensive disease. TCM diagnoses of headache and dizziness due to hyperactivity of liver- yang and asthenia of kidney-yin were made in the mean time.

Therapeutic principles of nourishing kidney- yin, calming the liver and suppressing the yang hyperactivity were performed.

Recipe:

tuber of elevated gastrodia, Rhizoma Gastrodiae 10g

chrysanthemum, Flos Chrysanthemi 10g

lucid asparagus root, Radix Asparagi 10g

ophiopogon root, Radix Ophiopogonis 10g

root-bark of peony, Cortex Moutan Radicis 10g

gambirplant, Ramulus Uncariae cum Uncis 12g

Chinese wolfberry fruit, Fructus Lycii 12g

herbaceous peony root, Radix Paeoniae Alba 12g

bidentate achyranthes root, Radix Achyranthis Bidentatae 12g

figwort root, Radix Scrophulariae 12g

shell of abalone, Concha Haliotidis 18g

selfheal spica, Spica Prunellae 15g

oriental water plantain rhizome, Rhizoma Alismatis 15g

dried root of rehmannia, Radix Rehmanniae 15g

oyster shell, Concha Ostreae 15g

licorice root, Radix Glycyrrhizae 5g

The dizziness was relieved after taking three doses

of the above recipe. The blood pressure decreased to
20. 0/12. 7kPa(150/95mmHg). The other symptoms
also improved. The blood pressure recovered to 18. 7/
12. 0k a (140/90mmHg) after taking over twenty
doses and the other symptoms disappeared. No relapse
was claimed at follow-ups in the subsequent two years.

CASE 6

Asthenia of the Liver and Kidney- yin Combined
with Hyperactivity of Liver-yang

Zeng, a 57-year-old female, worker, came to the
hospital on account of constant dizziness with a history
of hypertension for more than ten years.

The patient was found to be concerned with hypertension 10 years previously. From then on, she often complained of dizziness and light- headedness, tinnitus, palpitation, and insomnia. The blood pressure
had been as high as 25. 3/18. 1kPa (190/130mmHg).

On examination, the tongue was thin with little
fur; deep, thready and rapid pulse. The blood pressure
was 22. 1/16. 8kPa(166/126mmHg).

A TCM diagnosis of dizziness due to asthenia of
liver and kidney- yin and hyperactivity of liver-yang

was made.

Therapeutic principles of nourishing both kidney and liver- yin, calming the liver and suppressing the yang hyperactivity were performed.

Recipe:

prepared rhizome of rehmannia, Rhizoma Rehmanniae Praeparata 20g

Chinese yam rhizome, Rhizoma Dioscoreae 20g

fruit of Chinese wolfberry, Fructus Lycii 20g

bidentate achyranthes root, Radix Achyranthis Bidentatae 20g

root of herbaceous peony, Radix Paeoniae Alba 20g

root of red rooted salvia, Radix Salviae Miltiorrhizae 20g

poria, Poria 15g

oriental water plantain rhizome, Rhizoma Alismatis 15g

chrysanthemum, Flos Chrysanthemi 15g

root-bark of peony, Cortex Moutan Radicis 10g

Chinese date, Fructus Ziziphi Jujubae 10g

oyster shell, Concha Ostreae 30g

The blood pressure was lowered to 19. 5/13. 3kPa (146/100mmHg) after taking 5 doses of the above recipe. Fruit of glossy privet (Fructus Ligustri Lucidi) 20g and tuber of multiflower knotweed (Radix Polygoni Multiflori) 20g were added to the former recipe. After taking the other 15 doses the blood pressure decreased to 17. 3/11. 2kPa (130/84mmHg). The blood pressure remained normal and no relapse was claimed at follow- ups in the subsequent two years.

CASE 7

Liver-wind Stirring Inside(Asthenic Type)

A 72-year-old female, was admitted to the hospital on account of high blood pressure and recent facial hemiparalysis.

The patient had had an attack of cerebrovascular accident which led to hemiparalysis. She complained of dizziness which was severe in the afternoon, deviation of the left eye and mouth, insomnia and dreaminess, numbness of the extremities.

On examination, the patient was a normal nourished woman of thin build. The tongue was red with thin yellow fur. The pulse was taut and slippery. The blood pressure was 25. 6/13. 6kPa (192/102mmHg).

A TCM diagnosis of dizziness due to acute hyperactivity of liver-yang leading to liver- wind was made.

Therapeutic principles of calming the liver and suppressing the yang hyperactivity to stop liver-wind were performed.

Recipe:

powder of antelope horn, Cornu Antelopis 1. 2g

root of herbaceous peony, Radix Paeoniae Alba 15g

larva of a silkworm with batrytis, Bombys Batryticatus 15g

chrysanthemum, Flos Chrysanthemi 15g

gambirplant, Ramulus Uncariae Cum Uncis 15g

pearl shell, Concha Margaritifera Usta 30g

turtle shell, Carapax Trionycis 30g

root-bark of peony, Cortex Moutan Radicis 10g

dried root of rehmannia, Radix Rehmanniae 12g

The dizziness was alleviated in a considerable degree and the blood pressure decreased to 22. 1/12. 8kPa (166/96mmHg) after taking 3 doses of the above recipe. The dizziness was relieved and the facial hemiparalysis was removed several days later. The blood pressure recovered to normal. Qi Ju Dihuang Wan(Bolus of Six Drugs, Rehmannia with Wolfberry and Chrysanthemum) was used to strengthen the therapeutic effects.

CASE 8

Liver-wind Stirring Inside Combined with Phlegm- Heat

Cao, a 76-year-old male, was admitted to our hospital on account of hemiparalysis of the right extremities and mental confusion that began one week earlier.

The patient had a history of hypertension and cerebral ateriosclerosis for many years. He was fairly well until one morning a week before entry, when he had an accident of falling to the ground leading to unconsciousness and hemiparalysis of the right extremities. The patient was thus admitted to a hospital. He was diagnosed cerebral hemorrhage and tertiary hypertension by that hospital. Treatment of several kinds such as dehydralyzing, and oxygen therapy failed to take favorable effects. The patient was then admitted to our hospital. He had suffered from constipation for 3 days.

Examination revealed flushing, violent snoring, rale produced by the collection of sputum, deviation of the eye and mouth, aphasia, incontinence of urine, yellow tongue fur, slippery and rapid pulse. The blood pressure was 25. 3/16. 0kPa(190/120mmHg).

A diagnosis of apoplexy due to liver- wind and phlegm-heat stirring inside was made.

Therapeutic principles of calming the liver, and resolving phlegm-heat were performed.

Recipe:

antelope horn, Cornu Antelopis 5g

gambirplant, Ramulus Uncariae Cum Uncis 15g

pinellia(tuber), Rhizoma Pinelliae 10g

poria, Poria 10g

dried orange peel, Pericarpium Citri Reticulatae 10g

fruit of immature citron, Fructus Aurantii Immaturus 10g

bamboo shavings, Caulis Bambusae in Taeniam 10g

grass-leaved sweetflag, Rhizoma Acori Graminei 10g

rhubarb root, Radix et Rhizoma Rhei 12g

bidentate achyranthes root, Radix Achyranthis Bidentatae 12g

After taking 3 doses of the above decoction, the

constipation was removed and the consciousness improved. However, the symptom of aphasia still existed. Radix et Rhizoma Rhei was discharged from the former recipe and Lumbricus was added. After taking the other 10 doses of the decoction the patient was able to do some simple exercises except that the right hand could not hold anything. The blood pressure was 22. 1/ 12. 8kPa （166/96mmHg）. The patient was able to walk with the help of a stick one month later. The blood pressure was 22. 1/12. 0kPa（166/90mmHg）. A recipe consists of root of red rooted salvia（Radix Salviae Miltiorrhizae） , bidentate achyranthes root（Radix Achyranthis Bidentatae） , earthworm （Lumbricus）, gambirplant（Ramulus Uncariae cum Uncis）, motherwort fruit（Herba Leonuri）, pearl shell（Chocha Margaritifera Usta）, bark of eucommia （Cortex Eucommiae） was given orally to the patient one dose daily in the subsequent half one year. The blood pressure recovered to normal and he was discharged.

CASE 9

Liver-wind Stirring Inside （Asthenic Type ）
Zhang, a 91-year-old male, was admitted to the hospi-

tal on account of severe dizziness and numbness of both hands that began one day earlier.

The patient had a history of hypertension of over twenty years' duration. Hypotensors had been constantly given to control the condition. Last night he began to suffer from the onset of severe dizziness accompanied with aphasia, numbness of both hands, obtuse reaction, fatigue of the lower extremities, akinesia, cold feet, constipation of two days' duration, and dry mouth.

Examination revealed flushing, purplish tongue proper with no fur, weak pulse. The blood pressure was 33. 3/18. 7kPa(250/140mmHg).

Differentiation: The symptoms were due to insufficiency of the kidney- yin leading to abnormal rising of asthenic yang. Cerebrovascular accident should be prevented first of all.

Therapeutic principle of nourishing kidney- yin to control the ascending asthenic yang was performed.

Recipe:

dried root of rehmannia, Radix Rehmanniae 30g

prepared rhizome of rehmannia, Rhizoma Rehmanniae Praeparata 30g

fruit of medicinal cornel, Fructus Corni 30g

fossil fragments, Os Draconis 30g

oyster shell, Concha Ostreae 30g

stem of noble dendrobium, Herba Dendrobii 10g

tuber of dwarf lilyturf, Radix Ophiopogonis 10g

fruit of Chinese magnoliavine, Fructus Schisandrae 10g

saline cistanche, Herba Cistanchis 10g

fruit of Chinese wolfberry, Fructus Lycii 10g

mankshood root, Radix Aconiti Praeparata 10g

ginseng root, Radix Ginseng 20g

root of narrow-leaved polygala, Radix Polygalae 5g

drug sweetflag rhizome, Rhizoma Acori Calami 5g

bark of Chinese cassia tree, Cortex Cinnamomi 5g

After taking one dose of the above decoction, the symptoms improved. The feet became warm and the flushing was relieved. The patient was able to speak with difficulty. The pulse was weak. After taking the other two doses the numbness of the hands was relieved. The patient could speak clearly. The tongue revealed red proper with thin white fur. The pulse was slow and thready. The lower extremities became stronger. However, there was difficulty in walking. The blood pressure was 26. 7/12. 3kPa（200/92 mmHg). Treatment was applied daily in the subsequent two days. In the end the blood pressure recovered to normal and the conditions improved. He was then discharged.

CASE 10

Deficiency of both Vital Energy and Yin

Xu, a 65-year-old male, came to the hospital on November 1st, 1990 on account of increased dizziness in the preceding half one month.

The patient had a history of hypertension of over twenty years' duration. He began to suffer from the onset of severe dizziness half a month previously, accompanied with soreness of the waist and knees, lassitude and fatigue, shortness of breath, palpitation, dry throat and mouth.

Examination revealed enlarged pale tongue proper with little fur, thready and weak pulse. The blood pressure was 23. 2/15. 7kPa(174/118mmHg).

A TCM diagnosis of dizziness due to deficiency of both vital energy and yin was made. Therapeutic principle of invigorating both vital energy and yin was performed.

Recipe:

milk veteh root, Radix Astrgali seu Hedysari 20g

dangshen, Radix Codonopsis Pilosulae 12g

poria, Poria 12g

Chinese yam rhizome, Rhizoma Dioscoreae 12g

fruit of Chinese wolfberry, Fructus Lycii 12g

oriental water plantain rhizome, Rhizoma Alismatis 12g

chrysanthemum, Flos Chrysanthemi 12g

gambirplant, Ramulus Uncariae cum Uncis 15g

prepared rehizome of rehmannia, Rhizoma
Rehmanniae Praeparata 15g

parasitic loranthus, Ramulus Loranthi 15g

fruit of medicinal cornel, Fructus Corni 10g

After 6 doses of the above decoction the dizziness was alleviated and the blood pressure decreased to 22. 1/13. 9kPa(166/104mmHg) . The patient recovered in a considerable degree. Tuber of dwarf lilyturf (Radix Ophiopogonis) 12g and fruit of Chinese magnoli-avine (Fructus Schisandrae) 10g were added to the above recipe. After taking other 12 doses all the symptoms were relieved and the blood pressure was lowered to 20. 5/12. 5kPa (154/94mmHg). The patient was told to take Sheng Mai San(Pulse- activating Powder, consists of ginseng, dwarf lilyturf tuber and Chinese magnoliavine fruit.) and Qi Ju Dihuang Wan(Bolus of Six Drugs, Rehmannia with Wolfberry and Chrysanthemum, consists of medicinal cornel, Chinese yam rhizome, root-bark of peony, oriental water plantain rhizome, wolfberry and chrysanthemum, prepared rhizome of rehmannia, poria.) as long-term treatment to strengthen the therapeutic effects.

CASE 11

Deficiency of both Kidney-yin and Yang

Zou, a 42- year- old male, came to the hospital on account of constant dizziness and light-headedness in the preceding several years.

The patient began to suffer from hypertension several years ago, when the blood pressure was generally as high as 20/13. 3kPa (150/100mmHg) . He complained of constant dizziness and light-headedness which could be aggravated by heavy labor, accompanied with soreness of the waist, tinnitus, aversion to cold, cold limbs, nocturia, impotence.

Examination revealed enlarged tongue proper with little fur, deep and thready pulse.

A TCM diagnosis of dizziness due to deficiency of

66

both the kidney- yin and yang was made.

Therapeutic principles of activating kidney- yang and nourishing yin were performed.

Recipe:

dried root of rehmannia, Radix Rehmanniae 30g

Chinese yam rhizome, Rhizoma Dioscoreae 30g

mankshood root, Radix Aconiti Praeparata 30g

fruit of medicinal cornel, Fructus Corni 24g

fruit of glossy privet, Fructus Ligustri Lucidi 24g

yerbadetajo, Herba Ecliptae 24g

fossil fragments, Os Draconis 24g

oyster shell, Concha Ostreae 24g

oriental water plantain rhizome, Rhizoma Alismatis 9g

poria, Poria 9g

root-bark of peony, Cortex Moutan Radicis 9g

cassia(twig), Ramulus Cinnamomi 9g

The decoction was given one dose daily.

20 days later the symptoms were relieved and the blood pressure decreased to 17. 3/10. 7kPa（130/80mmHg）. No relapse was claimed at a follow- up one month later.

CASE 12

Yang Deficiency of both Spleen and Kidney

Liu, a 50-year-old male, came to the hospital on account of recurrent headache which increased in the preceding half one year.

The patient began to suffer the onset of headache 7 years previously. It was so severe that it sometimes led to syncope. He was diagnosed primary hypertension by another hospital.

Treatment of various kinds had been used with no favorable effect taken. The blood pressure fluctuated between 26. 0/17. 3kPa and 20. 0/13. 3kPa (195 ~ 150/130~100mmHg). The patient then came to our hospital. He complained of dizziness and lightheadedness, parietal headache radiated to the nuchal region, aversion to cold, lassitude in loin and knees, nausea, poor appetite, loose stools twice to 4 times daily, diarrhea before dawn.

Examination revealed pale tongue proper with white fur, deep and thready pulse. The blood pressure was 24. 0/16. 0kPa(180/120mmHg).

A TCM diagnosis of headache due to deficiency of both spleen and kidney-yang was made.

Therapeutic principles of warming and invigorating the spleen and kidney- yang were performed.

Recipe:

prepared rhizome of rehmannia, Rhizoma Rehmannia Praeparatae 12g

bark of eucommia, Cortex Eucommiae 12g

fruit of malaytea scurfpea, Fructus Psoraleae 12g

Chinese date, Fructus Ziziphi Jujubae 10g

Chinese yam rhizome, Rhizoma Dioscoreae 10g

mankshood root, Radix Aconiti Praeparata 10g

bark of Chinese cassia tree, Cortex Cinnamomi 3g

fruit of Chinese magnoliavine, Fructus Schisandrae 3g

licorice root, Radix Glycyrrhizae 5g

nutmeg, Semen Myristicae 5g

evodia fruit, Fructus Evodiae 6g

ginger, Rhizoma Zingiberis Recens 3g

After taking 3 doses of the decoction, the headache was greatly alleviated and the nausea was relieved. His appetite improved and the stools recovered to normal. After taking the other 5 doses the symptoms of aversion to cold, headache and dizziness, diarrhea before dawn were all relieved. The pulse was normal and he became in full vigor.

Examination revealed the blood pressure 20. 0/11. 2kPa(150/84mmHg).

CASE 13

Deficiency of Spleen and Kidney-yang Combined with Stagnant Cold-dampness in the Stomach

Guan, a 52-year-old female, worker, came to the hospital on account of dizziness of 9 months' duration.

The patient was well until 9 months previously, when she began to suffer from dizziness. She had been to another hospital where she was diagnosed hypertensive disease and was given various kinds of treatment. However, the blood pressure was still no less than 24. 0/16. 0kPa (180/120mmHg). The patient then came to our hospital. She complained of dizziness, distending pain in the lumbar region, lassitude of the extremities, listlessness, poor appetite, ageusia, diuresis, loose stools, prolapse of uterus, excessive vaginal discharge, mild anasarca.

On examination, the patient was a well- nourished woman of fat build. The tongue proper was pale with white and greasy fur; the pulse was deep and weak.

A TCM diagnosis of dizziness was made. The

condition was due to spleen and kidney- yang deficiency along with cold-damp stagnated in the spleen and stomach leading to failure of yang- energy to ascend to the head.

Therapeutic principles of warming the spleen and kidney-yang, promoting the vital- energy and invigorating the spleen to resolve cold-damp were performed.

Recipe:

dangshen, Radix Codonopsis Pilosulae 20g

mankshood root, Radix Aconiti Praeparata 20g

Chinese atractylodes rhizome, Rhizoma Atractylodis 16g

dried ginger, Rhizoma Zingiberis 12g

pinellia tuber, Rhizoma Pinelliae 12g

katsumadai seed, Semen Alpiniae Katsumadai 10g

poria, Poria 10g

Job's tears, Semen Coicis 30g

Himalaya teasel, Radix Dipsaci 30g

licorice root, Radix Glycyrrhizae 3g

The drugs decocted in water for oral administration and given one dose daily.

After taking 5 doses of the above decoction, the symptoms were removed. Examination revealed red tongue proper with thin white fur, soft pulse. Blood pressure 18. 7/12. 0kPa (140/90mmHg). Semen Alpiniae Katsumadai was discharged from the former recipe and Radix Astragali seu Hedysari 20g was added. The other three doses were then given to the patient. After the above administration, the blood pressure recovered to normal. No relapse was claimed at follow-ups within the subsequent four years.

CASE 14

Deficiency of both the Spleen and Kidney- yang Combined with Retention of Water

Chen, a 37- year- old woman, came to the hospital on account of edema of the face and lower extremities of over two years' duration which increased in the preceding one week.

The patient began to suffer idiopathic edema over two years previously. She had a history of lumbago of two years' duration. The condition developed in the last one week, accompanied with dizziness, palpitation, lassitude, aversion to cold, and poor appetite.

Examination revealed pale tongue proper with thin white fur, deep, thready, and slippery pulse. Blood pressure 20. 0/13. 1kPa (150/98mmHg). Routine uronoscopy, liver function test and EKG were normal.

A TCM diagnosis of edema due to deficiency of both spleen and kidney- yang along with retention of water was made.

Therapeutic principles of warming and invigorating the kidney and spleen to resolve water retention and relieve edema were performed.

Recipe:

mankshood, Radix Aconiti Praeparata 6g

poria, Poria 30g

milk veteh, Radix Astragali seu Hedysari 30g

Job's tears, Semen Coicis 30g

large-headed atractylodes, Rhizoma Atractylodis Macrocephalae 12g

malaytea scurfpea, Fructus Psoraleae 12g

bark of eucommia, Cortex Eucommiae 12g

oriental water plantain, Rhizoma Alismatis 15g

Asiatic plantain seed, Semen Plantaginis 15g

bidentate achyranthes, Radix Achyranthis Bidentatae 15g

fangji, Radix Stephaniae Tetrandrae 9g

dried old orange peel, Pericarpium Citri Reticulatae 9g

The drugs decocted in water for oral administration and taken one dose daily. 3 doses consisted of one course of treatment.

After one course of administration the edema and lumbago were alleviated in a considerable degree. The blood pressure was lowered to 17. 3/10. 4 kPa (130/ 78mmHg). The following treatment was given to strengthen the effects. She fully recovered several months later.

CASE 15

Edema due to Yang Insufficiency

Xu, a 60-year-old male, came to the hospital on account of anasarca ann increased dizziness in the preceding half one month.

The patient had a history of hypertension of over ten years' duration. Hypotensors of various kinds had been given. However, the effects became poorer and poorer. Reserpinum and Magnesii Sulfas had been given to the patient for hypertensive crisis. he had taken great amount of traditional Chinese drugs in the preceding two years. 80 doses of a recipe nourishing kidney-yin and lowering asthenic yang were given to the patient in the last 5 months. Although the dosage was rather high, the blood pressure ascended to 32. 0/ 18. 7kPa (240/140mmHg) instead of recovering to normal. The patient then came to our hospital. He complained of distending pain in the head and dizziness, lassitude and listlessness, palpitation, anorexia, oliguria, and anasarca.

Examination revealed enlarged pale tongue proper with white, moist and glossy fur, taut, deep and thready pulse.

A TCM diagnosis of edema due to kidney- yang deficiency was made.

Therapeutic principles of warming and invigorating the kidney- yang to resolve edema were performed.

Recipe:

poria, Poria 50g

mankshood, Radix Aconiti Praeparata 30g

oyster shell, Concha Ostreae 30g

ginger, Rhizoma Zingiberis Recens 15g

root of herbaceous peony, Radix Paeoniae Alba 15g

tortoise plastron, Plastrum Testudinis 18g

bidentate achyranthes, Radix Achyranthis Bidentatae 20g

large-headed atractylodes, Rhizoma Atractylodis

75

Macrocephalae 20g

The drugs decocted in water for oral administration and given one dose daily. 3 doses consisted of one course of treatment.

After taking 3 doses of the above decoction, the symptoms of distending headache and dizziness were alleviated in some degree. Blood pressure 26. 7/ 16. 0kPa (200/120mmHg). After the other 4 doses' administration the urine increased and the other symptoms improved in a considerable degree. The blood pressure 25. 3/15. 3kPa(190/115mmHg). Poria was reduced to 20g. The subsequent 5 doses were given to the patient. He recovered with the blood pressure 21. 3/13. 3kPa(160/100mmHg) after the administration. The dosage of the recipe was reduced to 20 percent of the original and the new decoction was given to the patient 5 to 7 doses every month in order to strengthen the therapeutic effects. After 5 months' administration the blood pressure fluctuated between 20. 0/13. 3kPa and 22. 9/14kPa(150~170/100~105mmHg).

CASE 16

Ascending of Asthenic Yang due to Deficiency of Kidney-yin

A 42-year-old male, came to the hospital on account of hypertension of 5 years' duration and palpitation in the preceding half one year.

The patient began to suffer from hypertension 5 years earlier. He had been to another hospital where fluoroscopy of chest revealed left ventricular hypertrophy and diagnoses of arteriosclerosis and hypertensive cardiopathy were made. Treatment of various kinds had been given. However no favorable effect was taken. The patient then came to our hospital. He complained of headache and dizziness, light-headedness, distending pain in the chest, palpitation, dry throat, insomnia, soreness of the waist, morbid perspiration over the head accompanied with anhidrosis of the other regions, nocturia and diuresis.

Examination revealed red complexion, enlarged red tongue with thin white fur, taut and weak pulse.

Recipe:

prepared rhizome of rehmannia, Rhizoma Rehmanniae Praeparata 20g fruit of medicinal cornel, Fructus Corni 10g

bidentate achyranthes, Radix Achyranthis Bidentatae 10g

fruit of Chinese wolfberry, Fructus Lycii 10g

root of herbaceous peony, Radix Paeoniae Alba 12g

shell of abalone, Concha Haliotidis 15g

licorice root, Radix Glycyrrhizae 6g

mankshood, Radix Aconiti Praeparata 10g

bark of Chinese cassia tree, Cortex Cinnamomi 3g

The drugs decocted in water and given one dose daily. 5 doses' administration consisted of one course of treatment.

After taking 5 doses of the above decoction, the patient complained of increased dizziness. The other 5 doses of the same recipe were given subsequently. The dizziness and headache improved after the second course of treatment. Examination revealed fairly normal blood pressure. Shell of abalone was discharged from the recipe and 10 doses' administration of the new recipe were given orally to the patient in order to strengthen the therapeutic effects.

CASE 17

Deficiency of both Heart and Kidney-yang

Hu, a 66-year-old male, was admitted to the hospital on account of recurrent palpitation, shortness of breath and edema of the lower extremities that began two years earlier.

The patient began to suffer from recurrent palpitation, shortness of breath and edema of the lower extremities two years previously. He had been to another hospital where the symptoms were alleviated after some kind of treatment. The condition developed two years later. The patient was admitted to the same hospital. Examination revealed blood pressure 26. 7/17. 5kPa (200/132mmHg. Palpation revealed apex beat in the sixth spatium intercostale 2cm external to the left midclavicular line and positive result of ascites' sign. Stethoscopy revealed moist rales of the inferior part of the lungs. Diagnoses of hypertensive disease, hypertensive cardiopathy and third- degree heart failure. Treatment of various kinds failed to achieve favorable effects. The patient was then admitted to our hospital. He complained of palpitation, shortness of breath, cold limbs, and oliguria.

Examination revealed pale tongue proper with ecchymoses and moist white fur, deep and thready pulse.

A TCM diagnosis of edema due to deficiency of kidney and heart-yang was made.

Therapeutic principle of warming the asthenic yang to relieve water retention was performed.

Recipe:

mankshood, Radix Aconiti Praeparata 15g

umbellate pore fungus, Polyporus Umbellatus 15g

ginger peel, Exocarpium Zingiberis Recens 6g

oriental water plantain, Rhizoma Alismatis 15g

cassia, Ramulus Cinnamomi 10g

root of herbaceous peony, Radix Paeoniae Alba 15g

shell of areca nut, Pericarpium Arecae 10g

poria, Poria 20g

large-headed atractylodes, Rhizoma Atractylodis Macrocephalae 12g

The drugs decocted in water and taken one dose daily. Radix ginseng 15g and Radix salviae miltiorrhizae 15g decocted and taken frequently. Five doses consisted of one course of treatment.

Five days later, the urine increased and the edema was alleviated. The shortness of breath improved in some degree. After the subsequent 8 doses' administration the edema was relieved and the symptoms of palpitation and shortness of breath disappeared. The blood pressure decreased to 22. 7/12. 0kPa（170/90mmHg）. Shipisan（Powder for Reinforcing the Spleen）consisting of Cortex magnoliae officinalis, Rhizoma atractylodis macrocephalae, Fructus tsaoko, Pericarpium arecae, Radix aconiti praeparata, Radix glycyrrhizae, Rhizoma zingiberis, Rhizoma zingiberis recens, Fructus ziziphi jujubae and Poria was given to the patient as a long-term administration in order to strengthen the therapeutic effects.

CASE 18

Stagnation of Phlegm in the Interior

Jiao, a 49-year-old male, was admitted to the hospital on account of recurrence of hypertensive disease that began one month earlier.

The patient had a history of hypertension of 3 years' duration. The symptoms were relieved by another hospital. He began to suffer the recurrence of severe headache and dizziness one month previously. He was then admitted to our hospital. The blood pressure was abnormally high even after two weeks' treatment, accompanied with the symptoms of heaviness and distending pain in the head, chest distress and nausea. The patient was then admitted to the TCM department. He complained of distending pain in the chest and hypochondriac region, poor appetite, nausea, heaviness of the head, and lassitude.

On examination, the patient was a well-nourished man of fat build. The complexion was pale. The tongue fur was greasy and white. The pulse was slippery and soft.

A TCM diagnosis of headache due to deficiency of spleen-yang and stagnation of phlegm in the interior was made.

Therapeutic principles of reinforcing the spleen to resolve phlegm and calming the internal wind were performed.

Recipe:

pinella, Rhizoma Pinelliae 15g

tuber of elevated gastrodia, Rhizoma Gastrodiae 15g

dried old orange peel, Pericarpium Citri Reticulatae 15g

gambirplant, Ramulus Uncariae cum Uncis 15g

ochre, haematitum 15g

oriental water plantain, Rhizoma Alismatis 15g

large-headed atractylodes, Rhizoma Atractylodis Macro Cephalae 20g

Asiatic plantain seed, Semen Plantaginis 20g

poria, Poria 25g

larva of a silkworm with batrytis, Bombyx Batryticatus 10g

licorice root, Radix Glycyrrhizae 10g

amomum fruit, Fructus Amomi 10g

The drugs decocted in water for oral administration one dose daily. 5 doses consisted of one course of treatment.

Second visit: The headache was alleviated in a considerable degree. His appetite improved.

Another three doses were administered to strengthen the effects. No relapse was claimed at follow-ups within one month.

CASE 19

Stagnation of Phlegm in the Interior

Chen, a 56- year- old woman, came to the hospital on account of severe dizziness that began 10 years earlier.

The patient had a history of hypertension of over 10 years' duration, accompanied by dizziness, tinnitus, stiffness of nape, chest distress, distending pain in the epigastric region, aversion to wind, nausea, abundant expectoration, and dry stools.

Examination revealed pale dark tongue proper with thick and greasy fur; slippery and rapid pulse; blood pressure 22. 7/16. 5kPa(170/124mmHg) ; total cholesterol 236mg%, triglyceride 286mg%.

The patient was diagnosed primary hypertensive disease(dizziness due to stagnation of phlegm in the interior in traditional Chinese medicine).

Therapeutic principles of resolving phlegm, reinforcing the spleen and regulating the incoordination between spleen and stomach were performed.

Recipe:
oriental water plantain, Rhizoma Alismatis 12g
poria, Poria 12g
pinellia, Rhizoma Pinelliae 12g
gambirplant, Ramulus Uncariae cum Uncis 12g
lotus petiole, Petiolus Nelumbinis 12g
puncturevine, Fructus Tribuli 12g

Job's tears, Semen Coicis 12g

bamboo shavings, Caulis Bambusae in Taeniam 9g

fruit of citron, Fructus Aurantii 9g

ro t-tuber of aromatic turmeric, Radix Curcumae 9g

selfheal, Spica Prunellae 9g

chrysanthemum, Flos Chrysanthemi 9g

Chinese radish seed, Semen Raphani 9g

dried old orange peel, Pericarpium Citri Reticulatae 9g

ginger, Rhizoma Zingiberis Recens 6g

The drugs decocted in water for oral administration one dose daily.

One week later the patient felt healthier than before with the symptoms greatly alleviated. The blood pressure recovered to 17. 3/10. 7kPa (130/80mmHg) after two weeks' administration. Examination four weeks later revealed total cholesterol 200mg%, triglyceride 138mg%.

CASE 20

Deficiency of Vital Energy and Stagnation of Phlegm

Yu, a 54-year-old male, came to the hospital on account of dizziness and light-headedness in the preceding two weeks.

The patient had a history of hypertension of over two years' duration. The blood pressure fluctuated between 24. 0/14. 7kPa (180/110mmHg) and 20/12. 0kPa(150/90mmHg). He began to suffer from severe dizziness and light-headedness two weeks previously, accompanied with chest distress, nausea, lassitude and listlessness, discomfort in the epigastric region, poor appetite and hypomnesis.

Examination revealed enlarged tongue proper with greasy fur, taut and slippery pulse; blood pressure 22. 7/14. 7kPa(170/110mmHg).

A TCM diagnosis of dizziness due to deficiency of vital energy and phlegm retention was made.

Therapeutic principles of reinforcing the vital energy, invigorating the spleen and resolving the phlegm were performed.

Recipe:

milk veteh, Radix Astragali seu Hedysari 30g

dangshen, Radix Codonopsis Pilosulae 15g

poria, Poria 15g

cassia seed, Semen Cassiae 15g

fruit of hawthorn, Fructus Crataegi 15g

bean of white hyacinth dolichos, Semen Dolichoris
Album 15g

dried old orange peel, Pericarpium Citri Reticulatae 9g

pinellia, Rhizoma Pinelliae 12g

large-headed atractylodes, Rhizoma Atractylodis
Macrocephalae 12g

red ochre, Ochra 20g

round cardamon, Semen Amomi Cardamomi 6g

ginger, Rhizoma Zingiberis Recens 3g

licorice root, Radix Glycyrrhizae 3g

The drugs decocted in water for oral administration one dose daily. Five doses consisted of one course
of treatment.

Few effects were taken after 5 doses' administration. Another course was then given to the patient.
Five days later the chest distress, nausea and discomfort in the epigastric region disappeared and the other
symptoms were alleviated in a considerable degree. Examination revealed enlarged tongue proper with thin
greasy fur, taut and slow pulse; blood pressure 21. 3/
13. 3 kPa (160/100mmHg). Rhizoma Zingiberis Recens was discharged from the recipe and after the fol-

lowing 10 doses' administration, all the symptoms disappeared and the blood pressure decreased to 18. 7/12. 0kPa(140/90mmHg).

CASE 21

Phlegm-fire Disturbing the Heart

Li, a 65-year-old male, was admitted to the hospital on account of severe headache accompanied by vomiting that began one week earlier.

The patient had a history of hypertension of over 20 years' duration. He suffered from severe headache accompanied by vomiting, numbness of the extremities and vague mind. The blood pressure was 24. 0/18. 7kPa（180/140mmHg）to 29. 3/21. 3kPa（220/160mmHg）. A diagnosis of hypertensive crisis was made by another hospital where treatment of hypotensor, diuretic and calmative tranquilizer therapies failed to achieve favorable results. The patient was then admitted to our hospital. He said that the onset was due to a quarrel over something one week previously. The accompanying symptoms included constipation, oliguria and irritability, saburra.

On examination, the patient was poor- nourished

woman of thin build. The complexion was flushed, the tongue proper was red with yellow greasy fur. The pulse was slippery and rapid.

A TCM diagnosis of mental confusion due to phlegm was made.

Therapeutic principles of lowering the abnormally ascending fire and resolving the phlegm to calm the mind were performed.

Recipe:

rhubarb, Radix et Rhizoma Rhei 10g

skullcap, Radix Scutellariae 10g

agalloch eaglewood, Lignum Aquilariae Resinatum 10g

root-tuber of aromatic turmeric, Radix Curcumae 10g

wrinkled gianthyssop, Herba Agastachis 10g

pinellia, Rhizoma Pinelliae 10g

oriental water plantain, Rhizoma Alismatis 10g

seed of wild jujube, Semen Ziziphi Spinosae 15g

root of the narrow- leaved polygala, Radix Polygalae 15g

dried old orange peel, Pericarpium Citri Reticulatae 15g

poria, Poria 15g

Chinese angelica, Radix Angelicae Sinensis 15g

milk veteh, Radix Astragali seu Hedysari 30g

jack-in-the pulpit, Rhizoma Arisaematis 30g

licorice root, Radix Glycyrrhizae 6g

The drugs decocted in water for oral administration one dose daily.

Three days later, the patient was able to speak correctly with ease and he could take some soft food. The defecation improved to once or twice a day. However he was bothered by the symptoms of urinary incontinence.

Examination revealed pale tongue proper with yellowish fur, soft and slow pulse, blood pressure 18. 7/ 13. 3kPa(140/100mmHg). Rhizoma Dioscoreae 10g, Semen Cuscutae 10g, Fructus Ziziphi Jujubae 12g and Cortex Eucommiae 15g were added to the recipe. After 4 doses' administration, the patient was able to walk with help and his appetite improved in a considerable degree. The blood pressure recovered to 17. 3/13. 3kPa (130/100mmHg). The other symptoms were also alleviated.

CASE 22

Blood Stasis

Wang, a 44-year-old male, worker, was admitted to the hospital on April 9, 1979 on account of headache and dizziness that began ten years earlier.

The patient had a history of hypertension of over ten years' duration, marked by dizziness, headache, and chest distress. Hypotensors had been constantly given to the patient. However, the blood pressure fluctuated between 17. 3/13. 3kPa (130/100mmHg) and 24. 0/16. 0kPa(180/120mmHg). He was then admitted to our hospital.

Examination revealed dark purplish tongue proper with white and greasy fur, deep and thready pulse.

A TCM diagnosis of headache due to blood stasis was made.

Therapeutic principle of removing blood stasis was performed.

Recipe:

cassia, Ramulus Cinnamomi 10g

peach kernel, Semen Persicae 10g

safflower, Flos Carthami 10g

chuanxiong, Rhizoma Ligustici Chuanxiong 10g

unpeeled root of herbaceous peony, Radix Paeoniae Rubra 10g

milk veteh, Radix Astragali seu Hedysari 15g

root of red rooted salvia, Radix Salviae Miltiorrhizae 15g

leatherleaf milletia, Caulis Millettiae Reliculatae 15g

milk veteh seed, Semen Astragali complanati 15g

puncturevine, Fructus Tribuli 15g

rosewood, Lignum Dalbergiae Odoriferae 6g

The drugs decocted in water for oral administration one dose daily.

Three days later, the blood pressure decreased to 17.3/12.0kPa(130/90mmHg). After continuously administration in the subsequent 20 days, the blood pressure recovered to normal and the other symptoms disappeared. He was discharged on July 5, 1979. No relapse was claimed at follow- ups within one year.

CASE 23

Blood Stasis due to Yang Deficiency

Lin, a 46-year-old woman, came to the hospital on account of headache and dizziness of over one year's duration which increased in the preceding 3 months.

The patient began to suffer from dizziness and headache more than one year previously, accompanied with aversion to cold, cold limbs, numbness of the extremities, insomnia and palpitation. The condition developed in the last three months.

Examination revealed pale and darkish tongue proper with thin and greasy fur, deep and thready pulse; blood pressure 20. 0/13. 1kPa(150/98mmHg).

TCM diagnoses of headache and dizziness due to blood stasis caused by deficiency of kidney- yang were made.

Therapeutic principles of warming the asthenic yang to promote blood circulation and lowering the abnormal ascending yang to calm the mind were performed.

Recipe:

mankshood, Radix Aconiti Praeparata 9g

longspur epimedium, Herba Epimedii 9g

root of red rooted salvia, Radix Salviae Miltiorrhizae 9g

unpeeled root of herbaceous peony, Radix Paeoniae Rubra 9g

flower of Chinese scholartree, Flos Sophorae 9g

large-headed atractylodes, Rhizoma Atractylodis Macrocephalae 9g

poria, Poria 9g

seed of wild jujube, Semen Ziziphi Spinosae 15g

fossil fragments, Os Draconis 15g

oyster shell, Concha Ostreae 15g

bidentate achyranthes, Radix Achyranthis Bidentatae 15g

The drugs decocted for oral administration one dose daily. 3 doses consisted of one course of treatment.

The patient felt healthier after one course of administration with the symptoms of aversion to cold and dizziness greatly alleviated. Headache and palpitation were relieved. However, numbness of the extremities still existed. Examination revealed pale tongue proper with thin white fur, deep and thready pulse; blood pressure 18. 7/11. 7 kPa(140/88mmHg). Radix Aconiti 3g, Radix Aconiti Kusnezoffii 3g and Radix Codonopsis Pilosulae 9g were added to the recipe and 5 doses were given to the patient. After administration all the symptoms disappeared. Examination revealed pale reddish tongue proper, slow pulse; blood pressure 18. 7/10. 7kPa(140/80mmHg). Another 5 doses were given to the patient to strengthen the therapeutic effects.

CASE 24

Blood Stasis Combined with Water Retention

Hu, a 50-year-old male, came to the hospital on account of nocturnal paroxysmal dyspnea of 3 years' duration which increased in the preceding 2 months.

The patient had a history of hypertension of 14 years' duration. He began to suffer from the onset of nocturnal paroxysmal dyspnea 3 years earlier. The condition developed in the last two months. The patient was often awaked by the dyspnea and shortness of breath, accompanied with palpitation, cough, frothy sputum, and loose stools. He was forced to be in orthopnea position to improve the respiration.

Examination revealed enlarged pale tongue with white fur, deep, taut and slippery pulse; blood pressure 20. 0/13. 3kPa (150/100mmHg); mild pitting edema of the lower extremities. Fluoroscopy revealed inflammatory changes of the inferior lobe of the right lung and left ventricular hypertrophy. EKG revealed left ventricular hypertrophy and myocardial strain and

95

left anterior fascicular block.

Diagnoses of hypertensive disease, hypertensive cardiopathy and left heart failure were made.

Therapeutic principles of promoting blood circulation, resolving water retention, reinforcing the spleen-energy and warming the asthenic yang were performed.

Recipe:

root of red rooted salvia, Radix Salviae Miltiorrhizae 30g

poria, Poria 30g

Asiatic plantain seed, Semen Plantaginis 30g

Chinese waxgourd peel, Exocarpium Benincasae 30g

milk veteh, Radix Astragali seu Hedysari 24g

shiny bugleweed herb, Herba Lycopi 15g

oriental water plantain, Rhizoma Alismatis 15g

root-bark of white mulberry, Cortex Mori Radicis 12g

large-headed atractylodes, Rhizoma Atractylodis Macrocephalae 9g

cassia, Ramulus Cinnamomi 45g

licorice root, Radix Glycyrrhizae 3g

The drugs decocted for oral administration one

dose daily. 15 doses consisted of one course of treatment.

The condition improved half one year later with the blood pressure 20/10. 7kPa(150/80mmHg) . Another 15 doses were given to the patient to strengthen the therapeutic effect. On examination, the EKG and heart function improved with the data as follows: $Rv5 + Sv1$ recovered from 6. 5mV to 4mV, PEP/LVET from 59% to 55%, a/E-0 from 23% to 21%. Phonocardiogram recovered to normal after the treatment.

CASE 25

Blood Stasis Combined with Phlegm Stagnation

Zhang, a 56- year- old male, came to the hospital on account of headache of 14 years' duration which increased in the preceding one week.

The patient was found to be concerned with hypertension 14 years previously. He had been admitted to another hospital on account of concussion of brain due to an accident 14 years previously. From then on he experienced the onset of recurrent headache. The condition developed one week before he came to the hospital when one morning he suffered severe headache accompanied with aversion to cold. Two days later the symptoms of aversion to cold disappeared, the pulsatile headache was severe on the left which increased during night and could be alleviated after exercises, accompanied with salivary sputum, dry mouth with bitter taste.

Examination revealed pale red tongue proper with thin white and moist fur, strong and taut pulse; blood pressure 21.3/16.0kPa(160/120mmHg). Therapeutic principles of calming the abnormally ascending yang was performed.

Recipe:

fruit of Chinese wolfberry, Fructus Lycii 12g

chrysanthemum, Flos Chrysanthemi 12g

root of herbaceous peony, Radix Paeoniae Alba 15g

gambirplant, Ramulus Uncariae cum Uncis 15g

bidentate achyranthes, Radix Achyranthis Bidentatae 15g

dried root of rehmannia, Radix Rehmanniae 15g

white mulberry leaf, Folium Mori 10g

poria with hostwood, Poria cum Ligno Hospite 10g

chuanxiong, Rhizoma Ligustici Chuanxiong 10g

The drugs decocted for oral administration one dose daily.

The patient failed to receive any favorable effect after taking 5 doses of the above decoction. After thorough differentiation, another diagnosis of headache due to blood stasis and phlegm was made.

Therapeutic principles of removing blood stasis and resolving phlegm were performed.

Recipe:

peach kernel, Semen Persicae 10g

safflower, Flos Carthami 10g

chuanxiong, Rhizoma Ligustici Chuanxiong 10g

unpeeled root of herbaceous peony, Radix Paeoniae Rubra 10g

pinellia, Rhizoma Pinelliae 10g

dried old orange peel, Pericarpium Citri Reticulatae 10g

tuber of elevated gastrodia, Rhizoma Gastrodiae 10g

chastetree fruit, Fructus Viticis 10g

licorice root, Radix Glycyrrhizae 10g

poria, Poria 15g

musk, Moschus 0. 1g

The drugs decocted in water except Mochus drunk

after mixing it singly with water. The recipe given one dose daily.

After 5 doses' administration, the headache was greatly alleviated and he was able to have a sleep of 3 to 4 hours during night. Rhizoma Corydalis was added to the recipe. After another five doses' administration the headache was relieved and he had a good sleep of 6 to 7 hours. Examination revealed the blood pressure 17.1/12.0 kPa(128/90mmHg).

CASE 26

Imbalance between Heart-yang and Kidney-yin

Xu, a 39-year-old woman, teacher, came to the hospital on account of insomnia in the preceding several days.

The patient had a history of hypertension accompanied with palpitation, dizziness, tinnitus, soreness of the waist and insomnia. The symptom of insomnia developed in the last a few days, accompanied with list-lessness and feverish sensation in the chest, on which account she came to our hospital.

Examination revealed red tongue proper with little fur, thready and rapid pulse.

A diagnosis of insomnia due to imbalance between heart-yang and kidney-yin was made.

Therapeutic principle of keeping the heart-yang and kidney-yin in balance was performed.

Recipe:

Chinese goldthread, Rhizoma Coptidis 4. 5g

rhizome of wind-weed, Rhizoma Anemarrhenae 9g

tuber of dwarf lilyturf, Radix Ophiopogonis 12g

seed of wind jujube, Semen Ziziphi Spinosae 12g

dried root of rehmannia, Radix Rehmanniae 12g

magnetite, Magnetitum 30g

cinnabar, Cinnabaris 0. 4g

drug sweetflag rhizome, Rhizoma Acori Calami 12g

donkey-hide gelatin, Colla Corii Asini 6g

root of the narrow- leaved polygala, Radix Polygalae 6g

bark of Chinese cassia tree, Cortex Cinnamomi 2g

The drugs decocted in water and given orally one dose daily.

After 5 doses' administration, the symptoms were alleviated and the blood pressure decreased to 21. 3/12. 0kPa(160/90mmHg). Another 10 doses were given to the patient to strengthen the therapeutic effects and after that the blood pressure recovered to normal.

CASE 27

Incoordination between the Chong and Ren Channels

Li, a 48- year- old woman, came to the hospital on October 25, 1987 on account of increased headache and dizziness in the preceding one month.

The patient had a history of hypertension of two years' duration marked by headache, dizziness, listlessness, irritability, feverish sensation in the head, perspiration, insomnia, dreaminess, amnesia, soreness of the waist, cold lower limbs. The symptoms of headache and dizziness developed in the preceding one week. She had a history of amenorrhea of over half one year's duration. The scanty menses of dark color came last week.

Examination revealed pale tongue proper with thin fur, taut and thready pulse; blood pressure 22. 7/14. 7kPa(170/110mmHg).

A TCM diagnosis of headache due to incoordination between the Chong and Ren Channels caused by impairment of liver and kidney- essence and abnormal ascending of asthenic kidney-fire was made.

Therapeutic principles of invigorating the kidney to clear away the asthenic fire and regulating the function between the Chong and Ren Channels were performed.

Recipe:

curculigo rhizome, Rhizoma Curculiginis 10g

longspur epimedium, Herba Epimedii 10g

Chinese angelica, Radix Angelicae Sinensis 12g

Indianmulberry, Radix Morindae Officinalis 12g

rhizome of wind-weed, Rhizoma Anemarrhenae 12g

corktree, Cortex Phellodendri 12g

root-bark of peony, Cortex Moutan Radicis 12g

fossil fragments, Os Draconis 30g

oyster shell, Concha Ostreae 30g

shell of abalone, Concha Haliotidis 30g

root of herbaceous peony, Radix Paeoniae Alba 15g

cape jasmine fruit, Fructus Gardeniae 6g

The drugs decocted for oral administration one dose daily. 6 doses consisted of one course of treatment.

The blood pressure decreased to 20. 7/13. 3kPa (155/100mmHg) after the above administration. The symptoms such as headache, listlessness and irritability were alleviated in a considerable degree. Cortex Moutan Radicis, Fructus Gardeniae and Concha haliotidis were discharged from the recipe and Fructus Mori, Rhizoma Polygonati and Herba Leonuri were added. The following 12 doses were given to the patient. The symptoms were relieved and the blood pressure recovered to 19. 7/12. 5kPa(148/94mmHg) after the treatment.

Other Cases

Wang, a 50-year-old male who presented a 2-year history of hypertension which showed aggravation from emotional stress recently. He complained of headache, dizziness, fidgets, flushed cheeks, insomnia, dreaminess, and dark urine. He had red tongue with yellow coating, and wiry pulse. Blood pressure 210/130mmHg. Previous treatment of various kinds failed to take any satisfactory effect.

He was diagnosed essential hypertension due to hyperactivity of liver-yang.

Recipe:

Ochra Haematitum 30g

Os Draconis 30g

Concha Ostreae 30g

Concha Margaritifera Usta 30g

Ramulus Uncariae cum Uncis 30g

Radix Paeoniae Alba 15g

Radix Scutellariae 12g

Decoct these ingredients for oral administration. Take one dose daily.

Blood pressure was brought down to 22. 7/13. 3kpa(170/100mmHg) with a remarkable alleviation of the symptoms after six doses of this recipe. All symptoms disappeared and blood pressure dropped to 21. 3/12. 0kpa(160/90mmHg) after another six doses. Considering the fact that there was too much intake of heavy materials, Concha Margaritifera Usta and Ochra Haematitum were consequently replaced by Flos Chrysanthemi 12g and Radix Cyathulae 15g in the recipe, to be taken continuously for another twelve days. Follow-ups for a half year showed no relapse.

Sun, a 48-year-old male, came to the hospital, who had headache and dizziness for a half year with a

blood pressure of 22. 0/13. 3kpa (165/100mmHg).
Hypotensors failed to take any satisfactory effect. In
addition to his old symptoms, he recently complained of
tinnitus, dry eye, feverish sensation in the palms and
soles, fidgets, amnesia, lassitude in loins and knees,
insomnia, dreaminess, and listlessness. He had red
tongue without coating, and wiry, thready pulse.
Blood pressure21. 3/13. 3kpa(160/100mmHg).

The patient was diagnosed hypertension due to deficiency of liver-yin and kidney-yin.

Recipe:

Radix Rehmanniae Praeparata 15g

Rhizoma Dioscoreae 12g

Fructus Corni 9g

Cortex Moutan Radicis 6g

Poria 12g

Rhizoma Alismatis 9g

Fructus Lycii 12g

Radix Paeoniae Alba 12g

Fructus Mori 24g

Ramulus Uncariae cum Uncis 24g

Decoct these ingredients for oral administration.
Take one dose daily.

The patient experienced an alleviation of his symptoms and his blood pressure was brought down to 18. 7/10. 7kpa(140/80mmHg) with the administration of this recipe for sixteen days. Follow-ups for one year showed no relapse.

Section 4
Specialists' Clinical Experience

He Ren, Professor of Zhejiang College of Traditional Chinese Medicine

Patients with the symptoms and signs of dizziness, headache, flushed complexion, bitter taste, listlessness, constipation, oliguria, dry and yellow tongue coating and taut pulse should be treated according to the therapeutic principles of calming the liver and clearing away liver-fire; recipe which can lower the ascending liver-yang and nourish kidney and liver-yin are given to patients marked by dizziness, tinnitus, amnesia, insomnia, heaviness of the head, listlessness and irritability, red tongue proper and taut, rapid pulse; patients characterized by dizziness, palpitation, shortness of breath, lassitude in loins and knees, insomnia, diuresis, white tongue fur, thready and taut pulse are given the treatment of nourishing liver and kidney- yin associated with that of warming the asthenic yang; therapeutic principle of resolving the phlegm to relieve dizziness should be performed as long as the symptoms and signs of dizziness, headache, chest distress, nausea, white and greasy tongue fur, slippery fur occur.

The proved recipe consists of white mulberry leaf (Folium Mori), white mulberry branch (Ramulus Mori), chrysanthemum (Flos Chrysanthemi), selfheal (Spica Prunellae), gambirplant (Ramulus Uncariae cum Uncis), bark of eucommia (Cortex Eucommiae) and fruit of glossy privet (Fructus Ligustri Lucidi).

Tan Riqiang, professor of Hunan College of Traditional Chinese Medicine

In Mr Tan's opinion, primary hypertension is divided into three types in accordance with clinical presentations:

1. Hyperactivity of Liver-yang: Marked by dizziness, headache, listlessness and irritability, bitter taste, flushing, red tongue proper with yellow fur, strong and taut pulse. Therapeutic principles of clearing away liver- fire and lowering the ascending liver-yang are performed. Tianma Gouteng Yin (Decoction

of Gatrodiae and Uncariae cum Uncis) consists of Rhizoma Gastrodiae, Ramulus Uncariae cum Uncis, Concha Haliotidis, Fructus Gardeniae, Radix Scutellariae, Radix Cyathulae, Cortex Eucommiae, Lignum Pini Poriaferum, Herba Leonuri, Ramulus Loranthi, Caulis Polygoni Multiflori, given mainly for clearing away liver-fire; Zhen Gan Xi Feng Tang (Decoction for Suppressing Liver-wind) consists of Radix Achyranthis Bidentatae, Haematitum, Os Draconis, Concha Ostreae, Plastrum Testudinis, Radix Paeoniae Alba, Radix Scrophulariae, Radix Asparagi, Fructus Meliae Toosendan, Fructus Hordei Germinatus, Radix Glycyrrhizae, Herba Artemisiae Scopariae adopted mainly to lower the ascending liver- yang by nourishing liver and kidney-yin.

2. Phlegm-Heat in the Interior: Marked by dizziness and heaviness of the head, distention of the epigastric region, nausea, listlessness, insomnia, bitter taste, oliguria, yellow and greasy tongue fur, taut and slippery pulse. Therapeutic principles of clearing away heat and resolving phlegm are performed. Patients of fat build are given Gouteng Wen Dan Tang (Decoction of Ramulus Uncariae cum Uncis and the Other Six Drugs for Clearing Away Gallbladder-Heat) consists of

Ramulus Uncariae cum Uncis, Rhizoma Pinelliae, Caulis Bambusael in Taeniam, Fructus Aurantii Immaturus, Exocarpium Citri Grandis, Rhizoma Zingiberis Recens, Radix Glycyrrhizae; Lingjiao Gouteng Tang(Decoction of Cornu Saijae Tataricae and Uncariae cum Uncis given to patients of thin build, consists of Cornu Saijae Tataricae, Ramulus Uncariae cum Uncis, Folium Mori, Bulbus Fritillariae Cirrhosae, Caulis Bambusae in Taeniam, Radix Rehmanniae, Flos Chrysanthemi, Radix Paeoniae Alba, Lignum Pini Poriaferum, Radix Glycyrrhizae.

3. Deficiency of Liver and Kidney-Yin: Marked by dizziness and light-headedness, headache, tinnitus, lassitude in the loins and knees, dreaminess, nocturnal emission, red tongue proper with little fur, taut and thready pulse. Therapeutic principles of reinforcing the kidney and nourishing the liver are performed. Shouwu Yan Shou Dan(Longevity Pill of Caulis Polygoni Multiflori) given to the subtype liver-yin deficiency, consists of Caulis Polygoni Multiflori, Radix Achyranthis Bidentatae, Semen Cuscutae, Cortex Eucommiae, Folium Mori, Flos Chrysanthemi, Fructus Mori, Fructus Ligustri Lucidi, Herba Ecliptae, Semen Sesami Nigrum, Herba Siegesbeckiae; Jia Wei Qi Ju Dihuang

110

Wan (Modified Bolus of Lycii and Chrysanthemi and Rehmanniae Praeparata) for the subtype asthenic kidney-yin, consists of Fructus Lycii, Flos Chrysanthemi, Cortex Moutan Radicis, Fructus Corni, Rhizoma Dioscoreae, Rhizoma Alismatis, Poria, Radix Rehmanniae.

Chen Shusen, Chief Physician of No. 301 Hospital of PLA

1) Therapeutic principles of calming the liver and lowering the liver-yang associated with that of calming the heart and nourishing heart-yin are performed for the type of hyperactivity of liver-yang.

Proved Recipe:

Rhizoma Gastrodiae 10g

Radix Cyathulae 10g

Rhizoma Anemarrhenae 10g

Ramulus Uncariae cum Uncis 20g

Caulis Polygoni Multiflori 20g

Flos Chrysanthemi Indici 15g

Radix Scutellariae 15g

Poria 15g

Ramulus Loranthi 15g

Spica Prunellae 15g

Semen Ziziphi Spinosae 15g

Concha Haliotidis 30g

Radix Gentianae and Rhizoma Alismatis added for oliguria and conjunctival congestion;

Semen Cassiae and Radix Rehmanniae for constipation.

2) Methods of nourishing liver and kidney- yin and lowering the ascending yang are given to the type of yin deficiency and hyperactivity of liver-yang.

Proved Recipe:

Fructus Lycii 10g

Cortex Moutan Radicis 10g

Radix Achyranthis Bidentatae 10g

Flos Chrysanthemi Indici 15g

Radix Rehmanniae 15g

Rhizoma Alismatis 15g

Poria 15g

Ramulus Loranthi 15g

Radix Paeoniae Alba 15g

Concha Ostreae 15g

Os Draconis 15g

Fructus Corni 9g

Ramulus Uncariae cum Uncis 20g

Radix Polygalae and Semen Ziziphi Spinosae added

for insomnia and dreaminess;

Natrii Sulfas 4g and Calculus Bovis 0. 5g mixed with water for oral administration in case of severe insomnia and dreaminess;

Radix Salviae Miltiorrhizae, Rhizoma Ligustici Chuanxiong and Flos Carthami for precordial pain; Radix Puerariae and Rhizoma Ligustici Chuanxiong for stiffness of nape;

Herba Siegesbeckiae, Ramulus Mori and Lumbricus for numbness of the extremities;

Radix Stephaniae Tetrandrae, Poria and Thallus Laminariae seu Eckloniae for edema of the lower extremities.

Methods of nourishing kidney- yin and reinforcing kidney-yang, calming the liver and promoting blood circulation are given for the type of deficiency of both kidney-yin and yang.

Proved Recipe:

Fructus Corni 10g

Rhizoma Dioscoreae 10g

Poria 10g

Cortex Moutan Radicis 10g

Rhizoma Alismatis 10g

Ramulus Uncariae cum Uncis 20g

Radix Rehmanniae 15g

Flos Chrysanthemi Indici 15g

Herba Epimedii 15g

Radix Salviae Miltiorrhizae 15g

Rhizoma Ligustici Chuanxiong 15g

Sargassum 15g

Cortex Cinnamomi 2g

Fructus Alpiniae Oxyphyllae and Fructus Psoraleae added for nocturia;

Radix Astragali seu Hedysari and Radix Codonopsis Pilosulae for lassitude;

Radix Ginseng, Radix Ophiopogonis and Fructus Schisandrae for chest distress, shortness of breath and palpitation;

Semen Ziziphi Spinosae and Rhizoma Anemarrhenae for restlessness and insomnia.

Calming the hyperactivity of liver- yang associated with nourishing heart-yin to calm the mind are of great importance to the treatment of hypertension. Drugs used to resolve wet- evil and promote blood circulation ought to be given to patients with refractory hypertensive disease.

Wu Songkang, Professor of Zhejiang College of

114

Traditional Chinese Medicine

Primary hypertension is clinically divided into 5 types: 1) hyperactivity pf liver- yang due to deficiency of both kidney and liver- yin; 2) hyperactivity of heart-yang due to deficiency of heart-yin; 3) deficiency of both kidney- yin and yang; 4) deficiency of both heart-yin and yang; 5) endogenous wind-syndrome. Treatment for the type of endogenous wind- syndrome is mainly discussed here. Hyperactivity of yang associated with yin deficiency or deficiency of both yin and yang may lead to the onset of endogenous wind- syndrome, which is marked by numbness of the face, extremities or tongue, muscular twitching and cramp, involuntary movement of limbs, or even distortion of the face.

Proved Recipe for Endogenous Wind-Syndrome:

Lumbricus

Rhizoma Ligustici Chuanxiong

Bombyx Batryticatus

Flos Sophorae Immaturus

Fructus Tribuli

Radix Scutellariae, Radix Rubiae, Fructus Gardeniae, Cortex Moutan Radicis added for convulsion, or even coma and high fever due to deficiency of liver and kidney-yin;

Radix Ledebouriellae, Ramulus Mori, Fructus Ligustri Lucidi and Herba Ecliptae for malnutrition of muscles due to deficiency of vital-energy and yin-essence;

Radix Astragali seu Hedysari, Radix Angelicae Sinensis, Semen Persicae, Flos Carthami and Radix Notoginseng for stagnant blood circulation due to blood stasis in the channels;

Rhizoma Coptidis, Rhizoma Pinelliae, Caulis Bambusae in Taeniam, Fructus Aurantii Immaturus, Exocarpium Citri Grandis, Rhizoma Zingiberis Recens, Radix Glycyrrhizae for phlegm retention; Fructus Aurantii Immaturus, Bulbus Allii Trichosanthis for yang deficiency accompanied with chest distress, chest pain radiating to the back, shortness of breath;

Rhizoma Anemarrhenae and Radix Angelicae Sinensis for incoordination between the Chong and Ren Channels.

Semen Celosiae 30g and Thallus Laminariae seu Eckloniae 20g are often added to the recipe. They are considerably effective for hypertension.

Zhu Guting, Professor of Zhejiang College of Traditional Chinese Medicine

Inspection of tongue plays an important role in the differentiation of hypertension.

Red tongue proper is the presentation of hyperactivity of yang due to yin deficiency. The following proved recipe is generally given to patients of this type:

Fructus Lycii

Flos Chrysanthemi

Cortex Moutan Radicis

Fructus Corni

Rhizoma Dioscoreae

Rhizoma Alismatis

Poria

Radix Rehmanniae Praeparata

Ramulus Uncariae cum Uncis

Concha Gardeniae

Radix Scrophulariae

Radix Ophiopogonis

Yin deficiency may cause insufficiency of intestinal juice, which will lead to constipation. It is one of the most commonly encountered symptoms of this type. Radix Rehmanniae, Radix Scrophulariae and Radix Ophiopogonis are most effective for dry stools and constipation. Dizziness and distending headache may favorably be alleviated after constipation has been relieved. The blood pressure may decrease in some degree in the mean time.

Hyperactivity of liver-fire is marked by dry and yellow tongue fur accompanied with dizziness and headache. The following recipe is given:

Radix Gentianiae
Radix Scutellariae
Fructus Gardeniae
Rhizoma Alismatis
Caulis Akebiae
Semen Plantaginis
Radix Angelicae Sinensis
Radix Bupleuri
Radix Rehmanniae
Spica Prunellae
Folium Mori
Concha Haliotidis
Flos Chrysanthemi
Ramulus Uncariae cum Uncis
Fructus Tribuli

Greasy tongue fur reveals the condition of phlegm retention and hyperactivity of liver-yang.

Proved Recipe:

Herba Agastachis

Cortex Magnoliae Officinalis

Rhizoma Pinelliae

Poria

Semen Armeniacae Amarum

Semen Coicis

Semen Amomi Rotundus

Polyporus Umbellatus

Semen Sojae Praeparatum

Rhizoma Alismatis

Ramulus Uncariae cum Uncis

Concha Haliotidi

Flos Chrysanthemi

The following recipe is administered in case of yellow and greasy fur:

Rhizoma Pinelliae

Caulis Bambusae in Taeniam

Fructus Aurantii Immaturus

Exocarpium Citri Grandis

Rhizoma Zingiberis Recens

Radix Glycyrrhizae

Poria

Herba Eupatorii

Ramulus Uncariae cum Uncis

Flos Chrysanthemi

Concha Haliotidis

Dizziness due to impairment of kidney- essence leading to hyperactivity of liver-yang is treated with the following recipe:

Radix Rehmanniae Praeparata

Fructus Corni

Poria

Rhizoma Alismatis

Rhizoma Dioscoreae

Cortex Moutan Radicis

Concha Haliotidis

Flos Chrysanthemi

Ramulus Uncariae cum Uncis

Folium Mori

Flos Chrysanthemi, Ramulus Uncariae cum Uncis and Concha Haliotidis Should be given to patients with hypertension of all types, in Zhu's opinion.

Lu Zhiqiang, Professor of Zhejiang College of Traditional Chinese Medicine

Primary hypertension is mainly due to hyperactivity of liver-yang, marked by dizziness, numbness, red tongue proper with yellow fur and taut pulse.

Proved Recipe:

Concha Haliotidis 30g

Spica Prunellae 15g

Ramulus Loranthi 15g

Flos Chrysanthemi 15g

Radix Scutellariae 9g

Radix Paeoniae Alba 9g

Radix Cyathulae 9g

Lumbricus 9g

Ramulus Uncariae cum Uncis 12g

Cortex Eucommiae 12g

Rhizoma Ligustici Chuanxiong 5g

Investigation showed that both diastolic and systolic pressure may be lowered 15 to 30 mmHg after administration of 15 doses.

Deficiency of both kidney-yin and yang may lead to hypertension marked by dizziness, soreness of the waist, lassitude of the lower extremities, pale red tongue, deep and thready pulse.

Proved Recipe:

Fructus Lycii 10g

Flos Chrysanthemi 10g

Cortex Moutan Radicis 10g

Fructus Corni 10g

Rhizoma Dioscoreae 15g

Rhizoma Alismatis 10g

Poria 6g

Radix Rehmanniae Praeparata 10g

Radix Achyranthis Bidentatae 9g

Radix Aconiti Praeparata 5 to 10g

Rhizoma Ligustici Chuanxiong 5g

It is favorably effective for the above type. Hypertension due to phlegm-fire is marked by distending headache and dizziness, poor appetite, cough with whitish and thick sputum, bitter taste, red tongue proper with white and thick greasy fur, or dry and darkish fur, slippery and taut pulse.

Proved Recipe:

Poria 12g

Caulis Bambusae in Taeniam 12g

Rhizoma Pinelliae 9g

Flos Chrysanthemi 9g

Radix Scutellariae 9g

Radix Achyranthis Bidentatae 9g

Herba Lophatheri 9g

Arisaema cum Bile 9g

Ramulus Loranthi 15g

Rhizoma Acori Graminei 3g

Exocarpium Citri Grandis 9g

Most cases received considerable effects after 7 doses' administration.

Wei Changchun, Chief Physician of Zhejiang Hospital of Traditional Chinese Medicine

Hypertensive disease belongs to the categories of hyperactivity of liver-fire, liver- yang and internal wind. The general therapeutic principle is to regulate the function of yin and yang. At the beginning of the onset, patient often complains of listlessness, irritability, bitter taste, headache, dry stools. Examination reveals flushed complexion, strong and taut pulse, red tongue proper with yellow fur, recurrent high blood pressure(often the systolic pressure). It is caused by abnormal rising of liver- fire. The following recipe is effective for this type:

Radix Scutellariae

Fructus Gardeniae

Radix et Rhizoma Rhei

Radix Paeoniae Alba

Radix Glycyrrhizae

Radix Rehmanniae

Ramulus Uncariae cum Uncis

Radix Achyranthis Bidentatae

Hyperactivity of liver-yang is marked by severe dizziness and light-headedness, listlessness, insomnia, lassitude of the lower extremities, flushed complexion, numbness of the face, red tongue proper, taut pulse, and high blood pressure (both the systolic and diastolic). It is commonly seen in prolonged cases.

Proved Recipe:

Flos Eriocauli

Spica Prunellae

Flos Chrysanthemi Indici

Ramulus Uncariae cum Uncis

Semen Cassiae

Lumbricus

Herba Ecliptae

Ramulus Loranthi

Radix Achyranthis Bidentatae

Impairment of kidney- yin is marked by light-headedness, palpitation, insomnia, numbness of the extremities, taut and thready pulse, dry and red tongue, high blood pressure(especially the diastolic). The proved recipe is as follows:

Fructus Lycii

124

Radix Rehmanniae Praeparata

Fructus Corni

Herba Ecliptae

Flos Chrysanthemi

Semen Cassiae

Ramulus Uncariae cum Uncis

Rhizoma Alismatis

Ramulus Mori

Radix Achyranthis Bidentatae

Complication of phlegm-fire is characterized by distending headache, dizziness, cough, shortness of breath, thick and yellowish sputum, slippery pulse, thick and yellow tongue fur. The following recipe is given to clear away heat and resolve phlegm:

Sargassum

Thallus Laminariae seu Eckloniae

Indigo Naturalis

Concha Meretricis seu Cyclinae

Radix Scutellariae

Fructus Aristolochiae

Semen Cassiae

Ramulus Mori

Cortex Mori Radicis

Deficiency of vital energy accompanied with

phlegm retention is marked by heaviness of the head, headache and dizziness, nausea, salivation, numbness of the extremities, deep and taut pulse, pale tongue proper with white fur. The following recipe is administered to warm the liver-energy, reinforce spleen and lower the adverse energy:

Fructus Evodiae
Radix Ginseng
Rhizoma Zingiberis Recens
Fructus Ziziphi Jujubae
Rhizoma Pinelliae
Semen Cassiae
Radix Achyranthis Bidentatae

Zhang Peiqiu, Chief Physician of Ningbo Hospital of Traditional Chinese Medicine

Liver and kidney are of vital importance to the onset of hypertension. Hyperactivity of liver- yang and yang-ascending due to yin-deficiency are commonly seen in clinic. The former is marked by dizziness and light-headedness, insomnia, thin tongue fur and taut pulse. The latter is Characterized by dizziness, heaviness of the head, tinnitus, dry mouth, listlessness, insomnia, red tongue proper, taut and thready pulse.

The following recipe is given to calm the liver-yang:

Rhizoma Gastrodiae

Ramulus Uncariae cum Uncis

Fructus Tribuli

Spica Prunellae

Flos Chrysanthemi

Rhizoma Alismatis

Concha Haliotidis

Concha Ostreae

Herba Siegesbeckiae and Ramulus Mori added for numbness of the limbs.

The following recipe is given to nourish yin and calm the liver:

Radix Rehmanniae

Fructus Lycii

Radix Polygoni Multiflori

Rhizoma Alismatis

Radix Scrophulariae

Fructus Ligustri Lucidi

Ramulus Uncariae cum Uncis

Concha Ostreae

Ramulus Loranthi and Radix Achyranthis Bidentatae added for soreness of the waist;

Semen Ziziphi Spinosae, Semen Biotae and Rhizoma Polygonati Odorati for palpitation and insomnia.

Deficiency of both yin and yang is usually seen in advanced stage, which is marked by dizziness, tinnitus, amnesia, numbness of the limbs, palpitation, shortness of breath, cold limbs and aversion to cold, lassitude of the lower extremities, nocturia or impotence, pale or red tongue proper with little fur, and thready pulse. The following recipe is administered to nourish yin essence and promote yang-energy:

Radix Rehmanniae Praeparata
Fructus Corni
Rhizoma Dioscoreae
Herba Epimedii
Radix Morindae Officicinalis
Cortex Eucommiae
Radix Achyranthis Bidentatae
Ramulus Loranthi

Radix Aconiti Praeparata and Cortex Cinnamomi added for severe yang deficiency marked by pale complexion, cold limbs and pale tongue;

Rhizoma Anemarrhenae, Cortex Phellodendri and Plastsum Testudinis for severe yin deficiency marked by listlessness, dry mouth, flushed complexion and red tongue proper;

Radix Astragali seu Hedysari, Rhizoma Atractylodis Macrocephalae and Radix Stephaniae Tetrandrae for vital energy deficiency marked by shortness of breath and facial edema. Tianma Gouteng Yin is effective for accelerated hypertension marked by severe headache, convulsion etc. . Cornu Saigae Tataricae 6g decocted singly is administered in case of hypertensive crisis.

Chen Zelin, Chief Physician of Zhongshan Hospital of Shanghai Medical University

Constipation is a commonly seen symptom of hypertensive disease. Radix et Rhizoma Rhei is most effective for constipation. In the mean time, it can also lower the blood pressure.

Cornu Saigae Tataricae should be administered constantly to prevent the onset of apoplexy, when symptom of numbness of the limbs and tongue occurs.

Deng Tietao, Professor of Guangzhou College of Traditional Chinese Medicine

Proved Recipes for Hypertension

Recipe 1. For hypertension due to hyperactivity of liver-yang.

Concha Haliotidis 30g

Concha Ostreae 30g

Radix Paeoniae Alba 15g

Radix Achyranthis Bidentatae 15g

Ramulus Uncariae cum Uncis 15g

Plumula Nelumbinis 6g

Stamen Nelumbinis 10g

Radix et Rhizoma Rhei added for constipation; Stamen Nelumbinis discharged and Poria, Rhizoma Alismatis added for thick and greasy tongue fur; Flos Chrysanthemi for headache due to heat-evil; Rhizoma Gastrodiae for severe dizziness; Semen Ziziphi Spinosae and Caulis Polygoni Multiflori for insomnia.

Recipe 2. For hypertension due to yin- deficiency of liver and kidney.

Stamen Nelumbinis 12g

Fructus Mori 12g

Fructus Ligustri Lucidi 12g

Herba Ecliptae 12g

Rhizoma Dioscoreae 15g

Radix Achyranthis Bidentatae 15g

Plastrum Testudinis 30g

Concha Ostreae 30g

Radix Ophiopogonis and Radix Rehmanniae added

for absence of tongue fur;

Radix Pseudostellariae for vital energy deficiency.

Recipe 3. For hypertension due to deficiency of both yin and yang

Ramulus Loranthi 30g

Stigma Maydis 30g

Magnetitum 30g(to be decocted first)

Os Draconis 30g(to be decocted first)

Radix Astragali seu Hedysari 30g, added in case of vital energy deficiency marked by enlarged pale tongue proper.

Recipe 4. For hypertension due to deficiency of kidney, especially the yang-energy.

Cortex Cinnamomi 3g

Rhizoma Polygonati 20g

Radix Aconiti Praeparata 10g

Fructus Mori 10g

Cortex Moutan Radicis 9g

Poria 9g

Rhizoma Alismatis 9g

Radix Achyranthis Bidentatae 9g

Stamen Nelumbinis 12g

Stigma Maydis 30g

Radix Astragali seu Hedysari 30g, Cortex Eucom-

miae 12g, Radix Paeoniae Alba 10g, Rhizoma Atractylodis Macrocephalae 10g and Rhizoma Zingiberis Recens 6g added for severe cases marked by edema.

Recipe 5. For hypertension due to phlegm retention caused by vital energy deficiency.

Radix Astragali seu Hedysari 30g

Haematitum 30g (to be decocted first)

Radix Codonopsis Pilosulae 15g

Poria 15g

Pericarpium Citri Reticulatae 12g

Rhizoma Pinelliae 12g

Semen Cassiae 24g

Rhizoma Atractylodis Macrocephalae 9g

Radix Glycyrrhizae 2g

Radix Polygoni Multiflori, Fructus Mori and
Fructus Ligustri Lucidi added for yin deficiency of kidney and liver;

Cortex Cinnamomi and Herba Epimedii for yang
deficiency of kidney;

Rhizoma Ligustici Chuanxiong, Flos Carthami,
Semen Persicae and Radix Salviae Miltiorrhizae for
blood stasis.

Shen Zhonggui, Chief Physician of Guang'an

Men Hospital of China Academy of Traditional Chinese Medicine

The following recipe is effective for hypertension due to abnormal rising of liver-fire:

Radix Rehmanniae

Radix Paeoniae Alba

Cortex Moutan Radicis

Spica Prunellae

Plastrum Testudinis

Concha Haliotidis

Flos Chrysanthemi

Herba Menthae

Pericarpium Papaveris

The above recipe can clear away liver- fire and nourish yin to lower liver-yang.

Hypertension due to hyperactivity of liver- yang is given the following proved recipe:

Folium Mori

Semen Sesami

Flos Chrysanthemi

Fructus Tribuli

Radix Polygoni Multiflori

Radix Rehmanniae

Radix Asparagi

Fructus Ligustri Lucidi

Radix Achyranthis Bidentatae

Semen Biotae

The above recipe has the effect of nourishing yin and calming the liver.

Therapeutic principles of nourishing yin and calming the mind are given to cases with hypertension due to yin deficiency (especially heart-yin) marked by dry mouth, listlessness, dreaminess, insomnia, thready and rapid pulse. The following recipe has such effect.

Radix Rehmanniae

Radix Paeoniae Alba

Herba Dendrobii

Semen Ziziphi Spinosae

Radix Polygalae

Poria cum Ligno Hospite

Os Draconis

Concha Ostreae

Caulis Polygoni Multiflori

Medulla Junci

Rhizoma Pinelliae

Rhizoma Coptidis

Cinnabaris

Radix Angelicae Sinensis

Radix Glycyrrhizae Praeparata

Hypertension partly due to deficiency of vital energy and blood is given the following proved recipe:

Folium Mori 9g

Flos Chrysanthemi 9g

Spica Prunellae 9g

Radix Astragali seu Hedysari 30g

Radix Rehmanniae 30g

Radix Linderae 6g

Lignum Aquilariae Resinatum 3g

Du Yumao, Professor of Shanxi College of Traditional Chinese Medicine

Primary hypertension is clinically divided into four types: 1) hyperactivity of liver- yang due to yin deficiency of both kidney and liver; 2) abnormal rising of liver-fire; 3)phlegm retention; 4)deficiency of kidney-yin and yang.

Hypertensive disease due to deficiency of kidney-yin and yang is marked by dizziness, tinnitus, amnesia, insomnia, palpitation, listlessness, lassitude, soreness of he loin and knees, edema of the lower extremities, cold legs, diuresis, massive vaginal discharge of dilute quality in woman cases, thin white tongue fur or

135

pale red tongue proper with no fur, deep and thready or taut pulse, recurrent high blood pressure. The condition should be differentiated from hyperactivity of liver- yang and abnormal rising of liver-fire. The following recipe is given to treat this type of hypertension.

Radix Rehmanniae Praeparata

Fructus Corni

Rhizoma Dioscoreae

Poria

Rhizoma Alismatis

Cortex Moutan Radicis

Ramulus Cinnamomi

Radix Aconiti Praeparata

Plastsum Testudinis, Radix Achyranthis Bidentatae, Radix Polygoni Multiflori and Carapax Trionycis added for severe yin deficiency marked by feverish sensation over the palms and soles, insomnia and flushed complexion.

Patients with climacteric hypertension are given the following recipe:

Rhizoma Curculiginis

Herba Epimedii

Radix Morindae Officinalis

Radix Angelicae Sinensis

136

Rhizoma Anemarrhenae
Cortex Phellodendri

Guo Zhiqui, Chief Physician of Xiyuan Hospital of China Academy of Traditional Chinese Medicine

Hypertension due to sthenic heat is commonly encountered in clinic. Drugs bitter in taste and cold in nature are effective for this type. Drugs used to replenish the vital essence are given in the mean time to prevent the side-effects such as impairment of vital essence and deficiency of stomach-yang which may occur after a long-term administration of drugs bitter in taste and cold in nature.

Drugs used to activate blood circulation are effective for hypertension due to stagnation of vital energy and blood stasis. These drugs are administered in high dosage especially to the persisting cases due to deficiency of vital energy and essence, stagnation of vital energy and blood stasis marked by dark purplish tongue proper, numbness of the extremities or chest pain. Hypertensive disease is generally due to hyperactivity of liver-yang and liver-fire, which may lead to endogenous-wind marked by numbness of the limbs or even convulsion. Drugs used to calm the liver such as Lumbricus, and Rhizoma Gastrodiae are administered as a prevention of apoplexy.

Li Zhongshou, Professor of Guangzhou College of Traditional Chinese Medicine

1) Hypertensive disease is caused by deficiency of liver, spleen and kidney.

Invigorating and nourishing vital essence and blood are of great importance to the treatment. He emphasized that drugs which nourish vital essence and blood should be given in high dosage. The following recipe is commonly administered :

Ramulus Loranthi

Radix Polygoni Multiflori

Caulis Spatholobi

Radix Rehmanniae Praeparata

Fructus Mori

Fructus Ligustri Lucidi

Fructus Lycii

Fructus Rosae Laevigatae

Semen Astragali Complanati

Cortex Eucommiae

2) The following drugs are effective for hyperactivity of liver-yang :

Concha Haliotidis and Concha Margaritifera Usta, which can clear away liver-fire and improve acuity of vision, are effective for the complication of hypertension such as visual disturbance, conjunctival congestion and photophobia, etc. ;

Concha Meretricis seu Cyclinae, used to clear away heat and resolve phlegm retention, is effective for thick and yellowish sputum due to lung-heat; Concha Ostreae, calming the mind and astringing the vital energy, is effective for palpitation, insomnia or nocturnal emission and night sweat. These drugs are administered 40 to 60g each.

3) High-dosage Radix Astragali seu Hedysari and Radix Ginseng are considerably effective for both hypertension and hypotension due to severe vital energy deficiency.

4) Blood stasis may be seen in clinic marked by dark purplish tongue proper with ecchymoses, chest pain and angina cordis etc.. It is caused by vital energy deficiency associated with yin or yang insufficiency. Radix Salviae Miltiorrhizae and Radix Notoginseng are the best to be selected.

5) Retention of liver-heat is commonly encountered in clinic marked by flushed complexion,

headache, bitter taste, throat pain, red tongue proper with yellowish fur. It belongs to the catagory of asthenic type. The following drugs are generally administered :

Flos Chrysanthemi, Spica Prunellae, Herba Ecliptae, Radix Puerariae, Cortex Mori Radicis, Caulis Bambusae in Taeniam, Radix Ophiopogonis, Flos Eriocauli, and Rhizoma Imperatae, have gentle effect to clear away liver-heat.

6) Drugs used to promote digestion are often administered to prevent heat-retention in the stomach which may cause ascending of blood pressure. The following recipe is generally given:

Cortex Magnoliae Officinalis

Fructus Aurantii Immaturus

Fructus Crataegi

Massa Fermentata Medicinalis

Fructus Oryzae Germinatus

Endothelium Corneum Gigeriae Galli

These drugs have the effect of both removing blood retention and promoting digestion.

Chapter Three
MATERIA MEDICA FOR
LOWERING BLOOD PRESSURE

Achyranthes and Cyathula Root
Radix Achyranthis
Bidentatae et Radix Cyathulae
Niu xi

ORIGIN   The root of Achyranthes bidentata, family Amaranthaceae.

NATURE,   TASTE   AND   CHANNEL TROPISM   Bitter and sour in taste, mild in nature, and attributive to liver and kidney channels.

EFFICACY AND INDICATION

1. Promote blood circulation to remove blood stasis, dredge the channels and oxytocic: For dystocia, retention of placenta, and blood stasis syndrome with amenia, dysmenorrhea, postpartum lochiostasis, abdominal pain, headache.

2. Ease the joint and strengthen bones, and muscles: For backache, pain and difficulty in movement of

the knees, flaccidity of extremities.

3. Induce the vital energy downward: For hyperactivity of liver-yang with headache, flaming-up of deficiency-fire with aphthae, toothache, hematemesis, epistaxis and hemoptysis.

4. Promote diuresis and relieve stranguria: For stranguria caused by urinary stone, stranguria of heat type and edema.

PHARMACOLOGICAL ACTION 1. Inhibiting the progress of experimental arthritis in animals, and antiphlogistic and antioncotic.

2. Its decoction or infusion induce contraction of gravid or ungravid uterus in experimental animals.

3. Its decoction exerts a transient hypotensive and diuretic effect.

DIRECTION Decoction: 6—12g.

Contraindicated for nocturnal emission, menorrhagia, collapse of middle-jiao energy and pregnant women. Radix Achyranthis Bidentatae is more effective for strengthening bones and muscles, and Radix Cyathulae is more effective for promoting blood circulation and removing blood stasis.

Antelope's Horn
Cornu Saigae Tataricae
Ling yang jiao

ORIGIN   The horn of Saiga tatarica, family Bovidae.

NATURE, TASTE AND CHANNEL TROPISM   Salty in, cold in nature, and attributive to liver and heart channels.

EFFICACY AND INDICATION   1. Clear away heat and calm the liver, expel wind and relieve spasm: For heat syndrome with convulsion, hyperactivity or wind transformation of liver-yang with dizziness, numbness and tremor of extremities and convulsion; for severe liver-fire syndrome manifested as epilepsy and insanity.

2. Chear away liver-fire to improve visual acuity: For conjunctivitis and and headache.

3. Clear away heat and toxic material: For febrile diseases with coma, delirium and mania.

PHARMACOLOGICAL ACTION   1. Intraperitoneal injection of its alcoholic extract exerts sedative effect in mice.

2. Its alcoholic extract and hydrolysate lower vac-

cine-induced fever in rabbits.

3. Analgesic, anti-convulsive and hypotensive.

DIRECTION　Decoction: 1—3g as slices decocted separately. Juice: 0.5—1.0g prepared by grinding.
Powder: 0.5—1.0g.

Aucklandia Root
Radix Aucklandiae
Mu xiang

ORIGIN　The root of Aucklandia lappa, family
Compositae.

NATURE, TASTE AND CHANNEL TROPISM
Acrid and bitter in taste, warm in nature, and attributive to spleen, stomach, large intestine and gallbladder channels.

EFFICACY AND INDICATION　Disperse the
stagnated liver energy and regulate the stomach, activate vital energy circulation and alleviate pain: For
stagnation of spleen energy and stomach energy with
fullness and pain in the abdomen, belching, nausea and
vomiting; for diarrhea and dysentery with abdominal
pain and tenesmus, used together with Rhizome Coptidis (Bolus of Aucklandiae and Coptidis); for stagna-

tion of liver energy and gallbladder energy with hypochondriac distension and pain, usually used together with Radix Bupleuri, Pericarpium Citri Reticulatea viride, Radix Scutellariae, etc. Also added to tonics in small dose for promoting digestion and regulation stomach energy.

PHARMACOLOGICAL ACTION 1. Dihydrocostus lactone isolated from its volatile oil relaxes the spasm of smooth muscles of bronchus and small intestine.

2. Its extract can lower blood pressure.

DIRECTION   Decoction: 3 — 9g (decocted later).

Bush cherry Seed
Semen Pruni
Yu li ren

ORIGIN   The seed of Prunus humilis or P. japonica, family Rosaceae.

NATURE, TASTE AND CHANNEL TROPISM   Acrid, bitter and sweet in taste, mild in nature, and attributive to large and small intestine channels.

EFFICACY AND INDICATION   1. Moisturize the intestine and relax the bowel: For constipation due to stagnation of large intestine or dryness of intestine, habitual constipation, etc.

2. promote diuresis and relieve edema: For edema, dysuria and beriberi.

PHARMACOLOGICAL ACTION   1. Diuretic and laxative.

2. Hypotensive.

DIRECTIONS   Decoction: 6—12g, crushed before decocting.

Capejasmine Fruit
Fructus Gardeniae
Zhi zi

ORIGIN   Fruit of Gardenia Jasminoides var. radicans, family Rubiaceae.

NATURE TASTE AND CHANNEL TROPISM   Bitter in taste, cold in natrue, and attributive to liver, lung, stomach and triple-jiao channels.

EFFICACY AND INDICATION   1. Purge sthenic fire to relieve vexation: For febrile diseases with irritability, insomnia, and even high fever, coma and delirium.

2. Clear away heat and promote diuresis: For jaundice and stranguria of dampness-heat type.

3. Clear away heat and toxic materials: For skin infection of intense heat type, erysipelas, burn and conjunctivitis.

4. Cool the blood and stop bleeding: For heat-syndrome with hematemesis, hemoptysis, epistaxis, hematuria, hemafecia, metrorrhagia, etc.

PHARMACOLOGICAL ACTION   1. The active components such as crocin, crocetin, genipin protect the liver from carbon tetrachloride and increase biliary secretion. Oral use of its decoction induce gallbladder contraction.

2. Oral or intraperitoneal use of its decection and alcoholic extract exerts a sustained hypotensive effect in anaesthetized and un-anaesthetized animals.

3. Hemostatic.

DIRECTION   Decoction: 3—9g.

Cassia Seed
Semen Cassiae
Jue ming zi

ORIGIN   Seed of Cassia obtusifolia or C. tora, family Leguminosae.

NATURE TASTE AND CHANNEL TROPISM Bitter in taste, slightly cold in nature, and attributive to liver and large intestine channels.

EFFICACY AND INDICATION   1. Clear away liver-fire and improve visual acuity: For liver-heat or wind-heat syndrome with redness, swelling and pain of eye, photophobia and lacrimation.

2. Suppress liver-yang: For hyperactivity of liver-yang or liver-fire with headache, dizziness, listlessness and bad temper, Recently used for hypertension.

3. Lower blood-fat: For hypercholesterinemia, hypertriglyceridemia and atherosclerosis.

4. Relax the bowels: For constipation due to accumulation of heat or dryness of the intestine.

PHARMACOLOGICAL ACTION   1. Oral administration of the herbal powder can inhibit the rising of serum cholesterol and formation of atherosclerosis in rabbits.

2. Its tincture and infusion can inhibit the myocardium of toad in vitro, and contract the blood vessels of lower limbs.

3. Its infusion can lower the blood pressure in dogs, cats, and rabbits.

4. Chrysophanol, one of the active components, is a laxative.

DIRECTION Decoction: 9—15g, crushed before decocting; 40—50g for lowering blood-fat.

Cat-tail Pollen
Pollen Typhae
Pu huang

ORIGIN   The pollen of Typha angustifolia, family Thphaceae.

NATURE,TASTE AND CHANNEL TROPISM Sweet in taste, mild in nature, and attributive to liver and pericardium channels.

EFFICACY AND INDICATION 1. Stop bleeding and remove blood stasis: For bleeding caused by trauma and blood-stasis, especially for metrorrhagia and menorrhagia.

2. Promote blood circulation to remove blood sta-

sis: For angina pectoria, postpartum abdominal pain, menalgia, abdominal pain and swelling and traumatic pain due to blood stasis. Recently used for hyperlipemia, especially for hypertriglyceridemia and hypercholesterinemia.

3. Promote diuresis and reduce stranguria: For stranguria complicated by hematuria and that of heat type. In addition, external use for exudative eczema.

PHARMACOLOGICAL ACTION 1. Strengthening the tone and promoting rhythmical contraction of uterus in animals and human.

2. Its decoction lowers blood pressure and shortens blood clotting time.

DIRECTION Decoction: 5 — 10g (wrapped with cloth). Powder: 2—3g, bid or tid. Tablet: 30g daily for coronary heart diseases and hyperlipemia.

Chuanxiong Rhizome
Rhizoma Ligustici Chuanxiong
Chuan xiong

ORIGIN The rhizome of Ligusticum chuanxiong, family Umbelliferae.

NATURE, TASTE AND CHANNEL

TROPISM   Acrid and bitter in taste, warm in nature, and attributive to liver, gallbladder and pericardium channels.

EFFICACY AND INDICATION   1. Promote the circulation of blood and vital energy: For stagnation of blood and vital energy resulting in angina pectoris, headache, chest pain, abdominal pain, dysmenorrhea, amenia, difficult menstruation or thromboangiitis obliterans.

2. Expel wind and alleviate pain: For recurrent headache, dizziness, headache of wind-cold type and rheumatism. Also used for leukocytopenia.

PHARMACOLOGICAL ACTION   1. Its active component, tetramethylpyrazine, can dilate the coronary artery and increase the coronary flow.

2. Its aqueous solution and alcoholic infusion can lower blood pressure.

3. Its alkaloids, ferulic acid and cnidilide are antispasmodics.

4. Inhibiting the growth of intestinal gram-negative bacteria and skin fungi.

DIRECTION   Decoction: 3 — 9g; 9 — 15g for serious cases. Tetramethylpyrazine injection: 40 — 120mg added in glucose solution IV in drips daily for angina pectoris and ischemic apoplexy. Sodium ferulate tablet: 10 mg tid for leukocytopenia and pectoris.

Cimicifuga Rhizome
Rhizoma Cimicifugae
Sheng ma

ORIGIN   Rhizome of Cimicifuga heracleifolia, C. dahurica and C. foetida, family Ranunculaceae.

NATURE, TASTE AND CHANNEL TROPISM   Acrid and sweet in taste, slightly cold in nature, and attributive to lung, spleen, large intestine and stomach channels.

EFFICACY AND INDICATION   1. Expel wind and hear, clear away toxic materials and let out skin eruption: For common cold of wind-heat type, and measles with indistinct eruptions, usually used together with Radix Puerariae.

2. Lift up yang-energy: For visceroptosis, used together with Radix Astragali seu Hedysari, and Radix Codonopsis Pilosulae.

3. Clear away heat and expel fire: For toothache due to stomach-heat, aphthae and headache, used together with Gypsum Fibrosum and Rhizoma Coptidis.

152

PHARMACOLOGICAL ACTION   1. Antipyretic, analgesic and anti-inflammatory. Gastric infusion of its extract (mainly containing ferulic acid) in a dosage of 1. 0g/kg can lower the body temperature of normal rats, and relieve the pain elicited by acetic acid in mice.

2. Inhibiting myocardium, slowing heart rate and lowering blood pressure.

DIRECTION   Decoction: 3—6g.

Coptis Root
Rhizoma Coptidis
Huang lian

ORIGIN   Rhizome of Coptis chinensis and C. deltoidea, family Ranunculaceae.

NATURE, TASTE AND CHANNEL TROPISM   Bitter in taste, cold in nature, and attributive to heart, liver, stomach and large intestine channels.

EFFICACY AND INDICATION   1. Clear away heat and deprive dampness from the middle-jiao: For diarrhea, dysentery and jaundice of dampness-heat type, stranguria of heat type.

2. Purge the sthenic fire and clear away toxic material: For various types of intense heat-syndrome, such as seasonal febrile diseases, sorethroat, conjunctivitis, burn, etc. Applicable to cases with high fever, extreme thirst, red tongue, yellow fur, rapid pulse, delirium and coma.

3. Clear away heart-fire and relieve vexation: For sthenic heart-fire syndrome with fever, chest upset and insomnia.

4. Purge sthenic fire to stop bleeding: For heat-syndrome with hematemesis, hemoptysis, epistaxis, hemafecia, or hematuria.

PHARMACOLOGICAL ACTION   Its chief component is berberine.

1. possessing broad-spectrum antibacterial and antiprotozoal effects.

2. Berberine exerts a hypotensive effect on experimental animals.

3. Small dosage of berberine enhances the action of acetylcholine on animals' hearts in vitro, while large dosage counteracts it.

4. Relaxing the smooth muscles of blood vessels and stimulating those of bronchus and gastrointestines.

5. Promoting bile secretion.

6. Berberine inhibits the cellular growth of ascitic cancer and lymphoma.

DIRECTION   Decoction: 3 — 9g. Tablet (berberine 0. 1 — 0. 2g): tid or qid.

Corn Stigma
Stigma Maydis
Yu mi xu

ORIGIN   The style and stigma of Zea mays L., family Gramineae.

NATURE, TASTE AND CHANNEL TROPISM   Sweet in taste and mild in nature.

EFFICACY AND INDICATION   1. Promote diuresis to relieve edema: For edema, ascites, wet beriberi, stranguria of heat type and that caused by urinary stone.

2. Promote choleresis and relieve jaundice: For hepatocellular jaundice, cholelithiasis and cholecystitis.

3. Lower blood pressure: For hypertension.

4. Lower blood sugar level: For diabetes mellitus.

5. Stop bleeding: For epistaxis, gingival bleeding. Recently, also used for thrombocytopenic purpura.

155

PHARMACOLOGICAL ACTION   1. diuretic.

2. Exerting significant and prolonged hypotensive effect.

3. Promoting biliary secretion and excretion.

4. Increasing the level of thrombocytes and thrombogen and promoting coagulation.

DIRECTION   Decoction: 15—30g.

Cow-bezoar

Calculus Bovis

Niu huang

ORIGIN   The gallbladder stone of Bos taurus domesticus (natural bezoar), or preparation derived from the gall of cow and pig (artificial bezoar).

NATURE, TASTE AND CHANNEL TROPISM   Bitter and sweet in taste, cool in nature, and attributive to liver and heart channels.

EFFICACY AND INDICATION   Clear away heat and toxic material, eliminate phlegm and wake the unconscious patient, expel wind and relieve spasm: For seasonal febrile diseases with high fever and convulsion, or with coma, delirium, lockjaw, abundant expectoration, red tongue, yellowish and greasy fur; for infantile convulsion, epilepsy and apoplexy; also for stagnation of heat-toxin manifested as sorethroat, skin infection and erosion, subcutaneous nodule, scrofula and breast carcinoma.

PHARMACOLOGICAL ACTION 1. Oral administration lowers experimental fever in guinea-pigs (200mg/kg) and in rats (300mg/kg).

2. Oral intake in a dosage of 600mg/kg/day for 6 days exerts an anticonvulsive effect.

3. Increasing biliary secretion.

4. Lowering blood pressure in rats with renal hypertension.

DIRECTION Pill or powder: 0. 15 — 0. 3g. External use: Appropriate amount.

Cyperus Tuber
Rhizoma Cyperi
Xiang fu

ORIGIN The rhizome of Cyperus rotunds, family Cyperaceae.

NATURE, TASTE AND CHANNEL TROPISM
Acrid slightly bitter and sweet in taste, mild in nature, and attributive to liver stomach channels.

EFFICACY AND INDICATION   Disperse the stagnated liver energy, activate vital energy circulation and alleviate pain, regulate menstruation and prevent miscarrige: For stagnation of liver energy with distension and pain of the hypochondria and breast, dysmenorrhea and irregular menstruation; for headache due to stagnation of liver energy; for those complicated by stomach-cold with epigastric pain, vomiting and acid regurgitation; for stagnation of liver energy and stomach energy with morning sickness and threatened abortion.

PHARMACOLOGICAL ACTION   1. Its 5% extract inhibits the uterine contraction in guinea-pigs in virto.

2. Analgesic.

3. Promoting the secretion of salive and gastric juice and expelling flatus.

4. Antipyretic. Its alcoholic extract lowers experimental fever in rats.

5. Slowing heart rate and lowering blood pressure.

DIRECTION   Decoction: 3—9g.

Dendrobium Stem
Herba dendrobii
Shi hu

ORIGIN   The stem of Dendrobium nobile, family Orchidaceae.

NATURE, TASTE AND CHANNEL TROPISM   Sweet and bland in taste, slightly cold in nature, and attributive to lung, stomach and kidney channels.

EFFICACY AND INDICATION   Nourish yin, clear away heat, benefit stomach and promote the production of body fluid: For febrile diseases with consumption of yin manifested as dry throat, thirst, asthenic-heat, and vexation; insufficiency of stomach-yin and flaming-up of asthenic fire manifested as epigastric pain, thirst, retching, red tongue with little coating or uncoated and smooth tongue.

PHARMACOLOGICAL ACTION   1. Dendrobine, one of its components, exerts the effects of raising the level of blood sugar, hypotensive, antipyretic and analgesic.

2. Its infusion is cardio-inhibitory.

3. Low dosage causes excitation while high dosage

causes inhibition of the intestine of rabbits in vitro.

DIRECTION   Decoction: 9—20g.

Dogbane Herb
Folium Apocyni Veneti
Luo bu ma

ORIGIN   Leaf of Apocynum venetum, family Apocynaceae.

NATURE,TASTE AND CHANNEL TROPISM
Bland and astringent in taste, cool in nature, and attributive to liver channel.

EFFICACY AND INDICATION   1. Calm the liver and clear away heat: For sthenia of liver-yang manifested as headache, dizziness, conjunctivitis, irritability and insomnia. Recently, used for hypertension.

2. Relieve cough and dyspnea: For cough of wind-heat type, chronic cough and dyspnea.

3. Promote diuresis: For edema and dysuria.

PHARMACOLOGICAL ACTION   Lowering blood pressure in dogs with renal hypertension.

In one study of dogs with perinephritic hypertension, their blood pressure was lowered from 25. 9/18.

9kpa（194/142 mmHg）to 20. 3/13. 3kpa（152/100 mmHg）two hours after oral administration of Dogbane herb，and it remained at a lower level for three days. No severe side effects were found，but weakness and dizziness occurred in some cases.

DIRECTION　Decoction：3—9g；may be used as daily drink.

Drink：3—6g per day.

Dutchmanspipe Fruit
Fructus Aristolochiae
Ma dou ling

ORIGIN　Fruit of Aristolochia contorta，family Aristolochiaceae.

NATURE，TASTE AND CHANNEL TROPISM Bitter and slightly acrid in taste，cold in nature，and attributive to lung and large intestine channels.

EFFICACY AND INDICATION　1. Lower blood pressure：For hypertension with heat-syndrome.

2. Clear away heat，relieve dyspnea，eliminate phlegm and relieve cough：For dyspneic cough of lung-heat type，cough of dryness-heat type with bloody sputum，and aphonia of lung-heat type.

161

3. Clear away heat in the large intestine: For hemorrhoids with pain and bleeding.

PHARMACOLOGICAL ACTION   Its decoction inhibits the growth of Staphylococcus aureus, Pneumococcus, Bacillus dysenteriae and dermatomyces in virto.

DIRECTION   Decoction: 3—9g.

Earth-worm
Lumbricus
Di long

ORIGIN   The body with the organs removed of Pheretima aspergillum or the whole body of Allolobophora caliginosa trapezoides, family Megascolecidae.

NATURE, TASTE AND CHANNEL TROPISM   Both are sour in taste, cold in nature, and attributive to liver, spleen and urinary bladder channels.

EFFICACY AND INDICATION   1. Clear away heat and calm the liver, expel wind and relieve spasm: For heat-syndrome with convulsion; for hyperactivity or wind transformation of liver-yang with dizziness,

162

headache and convulsion or manifested as epilepsy and insanity.

2. Relieve cough and asthma: For whooping cough and bronchial asthma.

3. Expel wind to alleviate itching: For urticaria, eczema and drug rash.

4. Expel wind to dredge the meridian: For arthralgia of wind-dampness-heat type, hemiplegia after apoplexy.

5. Promote diuresis: For heat-syndrome of urinary bladder with dysuria or retention of urine.

6. Lower blood pressure: For hypertension, especially that attributive to hyperactivity of liver-yang.

7. Oral and topical use may also be applicable in case of fracture, for relieving swelling, alleviating pain and promoting the growth of osteotylus.

PHARMACOLOGICAL ACTION   1. Relaxing bronchial spasm in rats or rabbits.

2. Intravenous injection of alcoholic infusion (0.1g/kg) lowers blood pressure in anesthetized dogs.

3. Sedative and anticonvulsive.

4. Lumbrifebrine, one of its active components, is an antipyretic.

DIRECTION   Decoction: 5—15g. Powder: 1—

2g bid or tid. External use: Appropriate amount.

Eucommia Bark
Cortex Eucommiae
Du zhong

ORIGIN   The bark of Eucommia ulmoides, family Eucommiaceae.

NATURE, TASTE AND CHANNEL TROPISM   Sweet and slightly acrid in taste, warm in nature, and attributive to liver and kidney channels.

EFFICACY AND INDICATION 1. Invigorate the liver and kidney, strengthen the tendons and bones: For deficiency of the liver and kidney manifested as soreness of the loin and knees, flaccidity of lower limbs.

2. Soothe the fetus: For threatened abortion due to hypofunction of the liver and kidney.

3. Lower blood pressure: For hypertension, especially those with deficiency of the liver and kidney.

PHARMACOLOGICAL ACTION   1. Hypotensive.

2. Promoting phagocytosis of mononuclear phagocytes.

164

3. Sedative and diuretic.

DIRECTION   Decoction: 9—15g; fried sample is better for hypertension.

Evodia Fruit
Fructus Evodiae
Wu zhu yu

ORIGIN   Nearly matured fruit of Evodia rutae-carpa, family Rutaceae.

NATURE, TASTE AND CHANNEL TROPISM   Acrid and bitter in taste, heat in nature, mildly toxic, and attributive to liver, spleen, stomach and kidney channels.

EFFICACY AND INDICATION   1. Disperse the depressed liver energy and alleviate mental depression, expel cold and alleviate pain, lower the adverse rising energy and stop vomiting: For stomach-cold syndrome with acid regurgitation and vomiting; for liver-cold syndrome involving the stomach with salivation and parietal headache; for incoordination between the liver and the stomach with hypochondriac pain, headache, epigastric and abdominal pain; colic of cold type, cold pain in the lower abdomen of women, beriberi of cold-dampness type with pain, etc.

2. Dry dampness: For pruritus vulvae and eczema.

3. Lower blood pressure: For hypertension. Also used for aphthae, infantile indigestion.

PHARMACOLOGICAL ACTION   1. Its volatile oil containing evoden inhibits the abnormal fermentation in the intestine.

2. Evodin, evodiamine and rutaecarpine, are active components for analgesic.

3. Oral administration or injection can lower blood pressure in normal animals or those with renal hypertension.

DIRECTION   Decoction: 3—9g. External use: powder prepared with vinegar.

Figwort Root
Radix Scrophulariae
Xuan shen

ORIGIN   Root of Scrophularia ningpoensis, family Scrophulariaceae.

NATURE, TASTE AND CHANNEL TROPISM   Sweet, bitter and salty in taste, slightly cold in nature, and attributive to lung, stomach and kidney channels.

EFFICACY AND INDICATION 1. Clear away heat, cool the blood nourish yin and moisturize dryness: For seasonal febrile diseases involving yingfen and xuefen with listlessness, thirst and eruptions, febrile diseases consuming yin with thirst, insomnia, constipation and dry, red tongue, lung-heat syndrome with dry cough or hemoptysis, diabetes, etc.

2. Purge the sthenic fire, clear away toxic material, soften the hard lumps and disperse the stagnation: For intense heat-syndrome or yin-deficiency syndrome with sore-throat, diphtheria, etc., usually used together with Radix Rehmanniae, Radix Ophiopogonis, Radix Scutellariae, Fructus Forsythiae; for subcutaneous nodes due to phlegm-fire, scrofula and goiter, used together with Bulbus fritillariae Thunbergii and Concha Ostreae.

PHARMACOLOGICAL ACTION 1. Its alcoholic extract and its component methoxycinnamic acid can lower the typhoid vaccine-induced fever in rabbits.

2. Its water or alcoholic infusion and decoction exert a mild hypotensive effect on anesthetized animals.

3. Lowering the level of blood sugar.

4. Its infusion inhibits the growth of some dermatomyces.

DIRECTION   Decoction: 9-30g.

Finger Citron
Fructus Citri Sarcodactylis
Fo shou

ORIGIN   The fruit of Citrus medica L. var sarcodactylis Swingly, family Rutaceae.

NATURE, TASTE AND CHANNEL TROPISM   Aromatic in odour. Acrid, bitter and sour in taste, warm in nature, and attributive to liver, spleen and lung channels.

EFFICACY AND INDICATION   1. Disperse the stagnated liver energy, activate vital energy circulation and alleviate pain: For stagnation of liver energy with distension and pain of the hypochondria and breast, dysmenorrhea or irregular menstruation, especially for those with insufficiency of liver-yin.

2. Regulate the stomach and strengthen the spleen: For spleen hypofunction and stagnation of vital energy with pain and fullness of the upper abdomen, and poor appetite.

3. Activate vital energy circulation and eliminate phlegm: For phlegm-dampness syndrome with productive cough and dyspnea.

PHARMACOLOGICAL ACTION   1. Its alcoholic extract relaxes the spasm of smooth muscles of gastrointestine, gallbladder and bronchus.

2. Its volatile oil is an expectorant and antiasthmatic.

3. Its alcoholic extract inhibits the heart and lowers blood pressure in anesthetized cats.

DIRECTION   Decoction: 3—9g.

Flower of Indian Dendranthema
Flos chrysanthemi Indici
Ye ju hua

ORIGIN   The capitulum of Chrysanthemum indicum, family Compositae.

NATURE, TASTE AND CHANNEL TROPISM   Bitter in taste, slightly cold in nature, and attributive to lung and liver channels.

EFFICACY AND INDICATION   1. Clear away heat and toxic material: For carbuncle, furuncle, skin nodules, scrofula and sorethroat, also for influenza.

2. Clear away liver-fire: For liver-fire syndrome with eye congestion, photophobia and lacrimation.

3. Hypertension with headache, irritability, and flushed face, wiry and rapid pulse.

PHARMACOLOGICAL ACTION   1. Yejuhua lactone or its flavone glycoside given orally, intraperitoneally or through the duodenum exert a hypotensive effect in unanesthetized rat and anesthetized cat and dog.

2. Inhibit the agglutination of blood platelet and promote the myocardial blood circulation.

3. Promote white cell phagocytosis.

4. Bacteriostatic.

DIRECTION   Decoction: 9—15g.

Flower of Magnolia
Flos Magnoliae
Xin yi

ORIGIN   The flower bud of Magnolia biondii Pamp., M. denudata Desr. and M. liliflora Desr., family Magnoliaceae.

NATURE, TASTE AND CHANNEL TROPISM   Acrid in taste, warm in nature, and attributive to lung and stomach channels.

EFFICACY AND INDICATION   Expel wind
and cold and clear the nasal passage: For sinusitis, allergic rhinitis, nasal polyp, hypertrophic rhinitis, etc.

PHARMACOLOGICAL ACTION   1. As an astringent to protect the nasal mucosa and as a vasodilator and antiphlogistic by improving blood circulation in the nose.

2. Hypotensive.

DIRECTION   Decoction: 3 — 10g.

Fritillary Bulb
Bulbus Fritillariae
Bei mu

ORIGIN   This drug has two variants: Sichuan
fritillary bulb and Zhejiang fritillary bulb.

Sichuan fritillary bulb comes from Fritillaria cirrhosa, F. unibracteata, F. przewalskii, or F. delavayi, family Liliaceae.

Zhejiang fritillary bulb comes from F. thunbergii, family Liliaceae.

NATURE,   TASTE   AND   CHANNEL
TROPISM   Sichuan fritillary bulb is bitter and sweet,

slightly cold, and Zhejiang fritillary bulb is bitter and cold. Both of them work towards lung and heart channels.

EFFICACY AND INDICATION   Resolving phlegm to stop cough and clearing away heat to dispel accumulation.

1. Sichuan fritillary bulb is sweet and cool and has the effect of moistening the lung. For cough, scanty sputum and dry throat due to deficiency of the lung, it is usually used with glehnia root and ophiopogon root. Zhejiang fritillary bulb is cold and bitter, and has a strong activity of clearing away heat to dispel accumulation. For cough due to affection by wind-heat exopathogens or due to stagnation of phlegm-fire, it is often used in combination with mulberry leaf and arctium fruit.

2. Zhejiang fritillary bulb is effective for scrofula, sores and abscesses. For scrofula, it is often used with scrophularia root and oyster shell, as in Scrofula-eliminating Pill (Xiaoluo Wan); for breast carbuncles, it is often used with dandelion and trichosanthes root; for lung abscess, it is often used with houttuynia and coix seed.

PHARMACOLOGICAL ACTION   Sichuan fritillary bulb, its active component fritimine can lower blood pressure, inhibit respiration, increase the level of blood sugar and stimulate the uterus in experimental animals.

Zhejiang fritillary bulb, intraperitioneal administration of its active components, peimine or peiminine, exerts a significant antitussive effect in mice.

DIRECTION Decoction: 3 — 10g, decocted in water for an oral dose.

Fruit-spike of Common Selfheal
Spica Prunellae
Xia ku cao

ORIGIN Spike of Prunella vulgaris, family Labiatae.

NATURE, TASTE AND CHANNEL TROPISM Bitter and acrid in taste, cold in nature, and attributive to liver and gallbladder channels.

EFFICACY AND INDICATION 1. Clear away liver-fire and calm the liver-yang: For hyperactivity liver-fire with conjunctivitis, photophobia, lacrimation and headache; for sthenia of liver-yang with dizziness, headache, irritability and bad temper. Recently also used for acute conjunctivitis and hypertension with the above manifestations

2. Eliminate phlegm and disperse stagnation: For subcutaneous nodule, scrofula, goiter and productive cough. Recently used for hyperthyroidism, thyroma, carcinoma of the lung and the esophagus, pulmonary tuberculosis, exudative pleurisy, icteric hepatitis, etc.

PHARMACOLOGICAL ACTION   1. Its decoction(100 mg/kg) for intravenous injection is hypotensive in dogs.

2. Its dilute decoction increases contractive power of toad and rabbit hearts in vitro, while concentrate decoction decreases.

3. Anti-inflammatory and bacteriostatic.

4. Adding the weight of adrenal cortex and promoting synthesis and secretion of corticosteroid in rats and in mice.

DIRECTION   Decoction: 6—12g, up to 30g.

Gastrodia Tuber
Rhizoma Gastrodiae
Tian ma

ORIGIN   The tuber of Gastrodia elate (Orchidaceae) symbiosis with Armillaria mellea, boiled with water or steamed and dried after the cortex is discarded.

NATURE, TASTE AND CHANNEL TROPISM   Sweet in taste, mild in nature and attributive to liver channel.

EFFICACY AND INDICATION   1. Calm the liver-wind: For syndrome of liver-wind stirring inside, such as infantile convulsion, tetanus, epilepsy, as well as dizziness and headache due to sthenia of liver-yang or the attack of wind-phlegm. Recently it is also used for the treatment of neurasthenia, nervous headache and hypertension.

2. Expel wind evil and alleviate pain: For migraine, arthralgia due to wind-dampness type, numbness of the extremities, and general fatigue, etc.

PHARMACOLOGICAL ACTION   1. Its active component gastrodin exerts as sedative, hypnotic and antispasmodic.

2. It may increase blood flow and decrease the peripheral resistance of blood vessels.

DIRECTION　Decoction: 3.—9g. Powder: 1.0—1.5g bid or tid.

Gentian Root
Radix Gentianae
Long dan cao

ORIGIN　The root and rhizome of Gentiana scabra,G. rigescens, family Gentianaceae.

NATURE,TASTE AND CHANNEL TROPISM Bitter in taste, cold in nature and attributive to liver, gallbladder and stomach channels.

EFFICACY AND INDICATION　1. Clear away heat and deprive dampness from middle-jiao: For jaundice, prurigo, vulvitis, leucorrhagia, etc. of dampness-heat type.

2. Purge the sthenic fire in the liver and gallbladder: For high fever with convulsion, sthenic heat-syndrome of liver and gallbladder, manifested as fever, headache, listlessness, hypochondriac pain, etc., usually used together with Radix Scutellariae and Fructus Gardeniae.

PHARMACOLOGICAL ACTION   Gentiopicrin and gentianine are the active components.

1. Oral administration of gentiopicrin can promote secretion of gastric juice and free hydrochloric acid and increase appetite.

2. Protecting liver and increasing biliary secretion.

3. Significant diuretic effect.

4. Anti-inflammatory effect of gentianine is $4-7$ times stronger than that of sodium salicylate.

5. Hypotensive.

DIRECTION   Decoction: $3-9g$.

Hawthorn Fruit
Fructus Crataegi
Shan zha

ORIGIN   Fruit of Crataegus pinnatifida and C. cuneata, family Rosaceae.

NATURE, TASTE AND CHANNEL TROPISM   Sour and sweet in taste, slightly warm in nature, and attributive to spleen; stomach and liver channels.

EFFICACY AND INDICATION   1. Strengthen

the stomach and improve digestion: For dyspepsia, especially over feeding in infants and immoderate eating of meats.

2. Relieve diarrhea and dysentery: Especially for those caused by immoderate eating and drinking.

3. Promote blood circulation and disperse blood stasis: For blood-stasis syndrome manifested as amenia, postpartum abdominal pain with lochiostasis, angina pectoris, polyp of vocal cord; also for inguinal hernia or swelling of testis with bearing-down pain, hepatosplenomegaly, and cystic hyperplasia of the breast.

4. Lower blood pressure and the level of blood lipids: For hypertension and hyperlipidemia.

PHARMACOLOGICAL ACTION   1. Its active component, triterpenic acid, increases coronary flow and improves systemic circulation.

2. Exerting prolonged hypotensive effect in anesthetized animals.

3. Counteracting the arrhythmias induced by pituitrin in rabbits.

4. Lower the level of serum cholesterol and β-lipoprotein in experimental animals with hyperlipidemia.

5. Digestant.

178

DIRECTION　Decoction: 6—12g; 30—60g for amenia, angina pectoris, polyp of vocal cord, hypertension and hyperlipidemia.

Herb of Common Cissampelos
Herba Cissampelotis
Xi sheng teng

ORIGIN　Herb of Cissampelos pareira L. var. hirsuta, family Menispermaceae.

NATURE, TASTE AND CHANNEL TROPISM　Sweet and bitter in taste, warm in nature.

EFFICACY AND INDICATION　1. Relax the muscles: Intravenous injection of cissampareine II as muscle relaxant for restoration of fracture.

2. Alleviate pain: for trauma and rheumatism.

PHARMACOLOGICAL ACTION　1. Its component cissampareine can block the autonomic ganglia, release histamine to cause hypotension.

2. Relaxing striated muscles.

3. Exerting cardiotonic effect on rabbits and frogs in vitro.

4. Stimulating the ileum of guinea-pigs in vitro.

5. Inhibiting the cells of nasopharyngeal carcinoma in vitro.

DIRECTION　Decoction: 9—15g.

External use: Appropriate amount.

Cissampareine II ampoule: 0. 25—0. 4 mg/kg IV.

Over-dosage of cissampareine II may cause respiratory failure, or even apnea.

Hemp Seed
Fructus Cannabis
Huo ma ren

ORIGIN　The fruit of Cannabis sativa, family Moraceae.

NATURE, TASTE AND CHANNEL TROPISM　Sweet in taste, mild in nature, and attributive to spleen, stomach and large intestine channels.

EFFICACY AND INDICATION　Moisturize the intestine and relax the bowels, nourish yin and restore vital energy: For constipation due to consumption of fluid and dryness of intestine; indicated for febrile disease with consumption of yin and fire hyperactivity, or yin-deficiency, consumption of fluid in the aged, as

180

well as postpartum anemia, also for habitual constipation.

PHARMACOLOGICAL ACTION   1. Laxative. Stimulating the intestinal mucosa, increasing secretion, decreasing water absorption and accelerating intestinal peristalsis.

2. Lowering the blood pressure in anesthetized cats and normal rats. Hypotensive for patients with hypertension after oral use for 5 to 6 weeks.

DIRECTION   Decoction: 9 — 30g (crushed before decocting).

Herb of Common Lophantherum
Herba Lophantheri
Dan zhu ye

ORIGIN   Herb of Lophantherum gracile Brongn., family Gramineae.

NATURE, TASTE AND CHANNEL TROPISM   Sweet in taste, cold in nature, and attributive to heart, stomach and small intestine channels.

EFFICACY AND INDICATION   1. Clear away heat and relieve vexation: For febrile diseases with fever, thirst and chest upset, usually used together with Gypsum Fibrosum, Rhizoma Anemarrhenae; for common cold of wind-heat type, used together with Flos Chrysanthemi, Herba Menthae, etc.

2. Clear away heart-fire and promote diuresis: For heart-heat syndrome with aphthae and oliguria with reddish urine, stranguria of heat type, usually used together with Caulis Akebiae, Radix Rehmanniae and Radix Glycyrrhizae.

PHARMACOLOGICAL ACTION   1. Antipyretic: Stomach perfusion of its infusion can reduce vaccine-induced fever in rats. The antipyretic effect of infusion (2g/kg) is 0.83 times as that of phenacetin (33mg/kg) in cats or rabbits.

2. Increasing the amount of chlorides in urine although its diuretic effect is weak.

3. Hypotensive.

DIRECTION   Decoction: 6—12g.

Herb of Glandularstalk
Herba Siegesbeckiae
Xi xiao cao

ORIGIN   Herb of Siegesbeckia orientalis and S.

pubescens, family Compositae.

NATURE, TASTE AND CHANNEL
TROPISM   Bitter in taste, cold in nature, and attributive to liver and heart channels.

EFFICACY AND INDICATION   1. Expel
wind-dampness and dredges the channels: For arthralgia of wind-dampness type, specially for wandering
arthralgia and those with swelling of joints, numbness
and immovability of extremities; also for apoplexy with
destortion of the face, aphasia, or hemiplegia.

2. Clear away heat and toxic materials, eliminate
dampness and relieve itching: For skin infection, jaundice of dampness-heat type, urticaria, eczema, psoriasis and pruritis.

3. Prevent the recurrence of malaria.

4. Tranquilize and lower blood pressure: For insomnia, neurasthenia, hypertension, used individually
or with Clerodendri Trichotomi.

PHARMACOLOGICAL ACTION   1. Hypotensive.

2. 1: 2 decoction of Herba Siegesbeckiae and
Clerodendri trichotomi inhibits the development of egg-
white induced arthritis in rats.

DIRECTION   Decoction: 10 — 15g, 30 — 45g

daily for malaria 2 — 3 hours before attack.

Immature Bitter Orange
Fructus Aurantii Immaturus
Zhi shi

ORIGIN The immature fruit of Citrus aurantium, family Rutaceae.

NATURE, TASTE AND CHANNEL TROPISM Bitter, acrid and sour in taste, slightly warm in nature, and attributive to spleen and stomach channels.

EFFICACY AND INDICATION 1. Activate vital energy circulation and eliminate phlegm, disperse stagnation and remove mass: For indigestion and stagnation of vital energy with feeling of fullness in the chest and upper abdomen, used together with Rhizoma Zingiberis, Rhizoma Coptidis; for phlegm-syndrome with productive cough and chest pain, used together with Fructus Trichosanthis, Rhizoma coptidis (Decoction for Mild Phlegm-Heat Syndrome in the Chest) for heat type and together with Pericarpium Citri Reticulatae, Rhizoma Zingiberis Recens for cold type.

2. Activate vital energy in the digestive tract: For stagnation of gastrointestine with diarrhea and dysentery with tenesmus, or constipation.

3. Supplement the vital energy: For hysteroptosis, gastroptosis, prolapse of rectum, etc. Recently, its injection is used for shock, and also effective for elevating blood pressure and improving blood supply of the heart, kidney and brain.

PHARMACOLOGICAL ACTION 1. Its active components, synephrine and N-methyltyramine, lower the blood pressure in anesthetized dogs.

2. Increasing the coronary flow significantly and heart rate slightly in anesthetized dogs.

3. Diuretic.

4. Its decoction inhibits the intestines in mice or in rabbits in vitro, stimulates the intestines in dogs with gastric fistula and intestinal fistula, and also induces contraction of gravid or non-gravid uterus in rabbits both in vivo and in vitro.

DIRECTION Decoction: 3—15g; 15—45g for visceroptosis.

Injection: For shock, 10-40g IV, followed by 20-100g IV in drips.

Large-leaf Gentian Root
Radix Gentianae Macrophyllae
Qin jiao

ORIGIN Root of Gentiana macrophylla and G. dahurica, family Gentianaceae.

NATURE, TASTE AND CHANNEL TROPISM Bitter and acrid in tsate, mild in nature, and attributive to stomach, liver and gallbladder channels.

EFFICACY AND INDICATIONS 1. Clear away heat, expel cold and dampness: For arthralgia of wind-dampness-heat type and muscular spasm.

2. Lower asthenic fever: For infantile malnutrition with fever, hectic fever due to yin-deficiency, usually used together with Rhizoma Anemarrhenae, Cortex Lycii Radicis.

3. Promote diuresis, relax the bowels, and relieve jaundice: For jaundice of dampness-heat type, dysuria ard dyschesia.

PHARMACOLOGICAL ACTION Gentianine is one of its active components.

1. Inhibiting experimental arthritis in mice and

186

decreasing capillary permeability.

2. Anti-allergic.

3. Inducing transient hypotensive effect.

DIRECTION Decoction: 6-12g.

Little Silver-banded Krait
Bungarus Parvus
Bai hua she

ORIGIN The whole body (viscera discarded) of Bungarus multicinctus multicinctus Blyth., family Elapidae.

NATURE, TASTE AND CHANNEL TROPISM Sweet and salty in taste, warm in nature, toxic, and attributive to liver channel.

EFFICACY AND INDICATION 1. Expel wind, dredge the channels, relieve muscular spasm: For rheumatism, especially the intractable cases and those with wandering arthralgia, numbness of the extremities and muscular spasm; also for apoplexy complicated by distortion of face and hemiplegia.

2. Relieve convulsive seizures: For infantile convulsion, tetanus and convulsion after apoplexy.

3. Expel wind and alleviate itching: For itching induced by scabies, tinea infection and urticaria.

4. Remove toxic materials: For leprosy, scrofula, and severe skin infections.

PHARMACOLOGICAL ACTION 1. Analgesic, sedative.

2. Hypotensive owing to its vasodilative effect.

DIRECTION Decoction: 3—10g. Powder: 1. 0—1. 5g.

Loranthus Mulberry Mistletoe
Ramulus Loranthis
Sang ji sheng

ORIGIN The branch and leaf of Taxillus chinensis or Viscum coloratum, family Loranthaceae.

NATURE, TASTE AND CHANNEL TROPISM Bitter in taste, mild in nature, and attributive to liver and kidney channels.

EFFICACY AND INDICATION 1. Expel wind-dampness and tonify the liver and kidney: For rheumatism with hypofunction of the liver and kidney manifested as weakness of back and knees and flaccidity of

188

extremities.

2. Nourish blood and calm the fetus: For threatened abortion due to hypofunction of liver and kidney.

3. Lower blood pressure: For hypertension, especially for those with deficiency of liver and kidney. Recently used for angina pectoris and arrhythmia.

PHARMACOLOGICAL ACTION 1. Lowering blood pressure in anesthetized dogs and cats by gastric infusion in a dose of 0. 4 — 0. 5g/kg.

2. Dilating coronary arteries and slowing heart rate.

3. Counteracting the exciting effect of caffeine.

DIRECTION Decoction: 10 — 30g. Instant granules: Half package (equivalent to 20g of crude drugs) bid. Ampoule (5 ml containing 10g of crude drugs): 10 ml added in 50% glucose Injection 20 ml IV once daily.

Lotus Plumule
Plumula Nelumbinis
Lian zi xin

ORIGIN The plumule or young leaf of Nelumbo

nucifera, family Nymphaeaceae.

NATURE, TASTE AND CHANNEL TROPISM Bitter in taste, cold in nature, and attributive to heart and kidney channels.

EFFICACY AND INDICATION Clear away heart-fire and relieve rexation: For hyperactivity of heart-fire manifested high fever, listlessness, coma, delirium, and insomnia, or hypertension with such manifestations.

PHARMACOLOGICAL ACTION 1. Its decoction can lower blood pressure.

2. Its alkaloids are cardiotonic.

3. Its component, demethylcoclaurine, may relax smooth muscles.

DIRECTION Decoction: 1.5 — 6.0g.

Lucid Ganoderma
Ganoderma Lucidum seu Japonicum
Ling zhi

ORIGIN The sporophore of Ganoderma Lucidum (Leyss. ex Fr.)Karst. or G. japonicum (Fr.) Lloyd, family Polyporaceae.

190

NATURE, TASTE AND CHANNEL TROPISM Both are bland in taste, warm in nature, and attributive to heart, spleen, lung, liver and kidney channels.

EFFICACY AND INDICATION 1. Tranquilize the mind, enrich vital energy and blood: For deficiency of heart energy or heart-blood manifested as insomnia, dreaminess, amnesia, dullness, frightening and severe palpitation; also used for all types of vital energy deficiency syndrome and blood-deficiency syndrome.

2. Eliminate phlegm, relieve cough and dyspnea: For deficiency-syndrome with cough and dyspnea. Recently also used for hyperlipemia, hypertension, coronary heart diseases, arrhythmia, leukocytopenia and hepatitis.

PHARMACOLOGICAL ACTION 1. Sedative and analgesic.

2. Increasing the tolerance of cold and anoxia in experimental mice.

3. Exerting mild and prolonged hypotensive effect in rabbits.

4. Protecting the liver of mouse from impairment and decreasing the level of SGPT (serum glutamic-pyruvic transaminase).

191

5. Decreasing the level of blood sugar.

DIRECTION Decoction: 3—10g.

Magnolia Bark
Cortex Magnoliae Officinalis
Hou po

ORIGIN The dried bark and bark of branch, root of Magnolia officinalis or M. officinalis var. biloba, family Magnoliaceae.

NATURE, TASTE AND CHANNEL TROPISM Bitter and acrid in taste, warm in nature, and attributive to spleen, stomach, lung and large intestine channels.

EFFICACY AND INDICATION 1. Activate circulation of vital energy, deprive dampness, keep the adverse energy downward and relieve dyspepsia: For abdominal distension and pain, nausea, vomiting, constipation or loose stool due to stagnation of dampness in the middle-jiao or indigestion and stagnation of vital energy. It is an important drug for relieving distension.

2. Calm the adverse rising energy and relieve dyspnea: For shortness of breath due to adverses rising of

lung energy.

PHARMACOLOGICAL ACTION 1. Broad-spectrum antibacterial.

2. Magnocurarine, one of the active components, can relax striated muscles, also lower blood pressure and accelerate heart rate.

3. Its decoction stimulates the smooth muscles of intestines and bronchi in rabbits in vitro.

DIRECTION Decoction: 3—9g (decocted later). Prolonged boiling will increase its toxicity.

Moutan Bark
Cortex Moutan Radicis
Mu dan pi

ORIGIN The dried bark of Paeonia suffruticosa, family Ranunculaceae.

NATUTE, TASTE AND CHANNEL TROPISM Bitter and acrid in taste, slightly cold in nature, and attributive to heart, liver and kidney channels.

EFFICACY AND INDICATIONS 1. Clear away heat and cool the blood: For eruptive febrile diseases, blood-heat syndrome with hematemesis, hemoptysis, epistaxis, etc., heat-syndrome consuming yin or yin-deficiency syndrome manifested as night fever, hectic fever and anhidrosis.

2. Promote blood circulation to remove blood stasis: For blood-stasis syndrome manifested as amenorrhea, menalgia, or abdominal mass, used together with Semen Persicae, Ramulus Cinnamomi, Poria, Radix Paeoniae Rubra (Bolus of Ramulus Cinnamomi and Poria); for periappendicular abscess, used together with Radix et Rhizoma Rhei, semen Persicae, Semen Benincasae, Natrii Sulfas (Decoction of Rhei and Moutan Radicis); also for skin infection, measles with incomplete and purple red eruptions.

Recently also used for allergic rhinitis.

PHARMACOLOGICAL ACTION Paeonol is one of its active components.

1. Antibacterial and anti-inflammatory.

2. Sedative. In mouse 125mg/kg intraperitoneally.

3. Analgesic. In mouse 1.0g/kg for gastric infusion.

4. Antipyretic. Reducing fever in mouse induced by typhoid or paratyphoid vaccines.

194·

5. Its decoction or paeonol can lower blood pressure in anaesthetized dogs and rats.

DIRECTION Decoction: 6—12g.

Notoginseng
Radix Notoginseng
San qi

ORIGIN   Root of Panax notoginseng, family Araliaceae.

NATURE, TASTE AND CHANNEL TROPISM Sweet and slightly bitter in taste, warm in nature, and acting on liver and stomach channels.

EFFICACY AND INDICATION Promote blood circulation to remove blood stasis, stop bleeding, relieve swelling and alleviate pain: For various kinds of bleeding due to trauma and blood-stasis syndrome, such as hematemesis, hemoptysis, metrorrhagia, hematuria, hemafecia and epistaxis, which manifested as dark petechia, localized pain, dull-coloured tongue with petechiae, etc. For amenia, menalgia, and trauma with blood-stasis syndrome. Recently also used for coronary heart disease, angina pectoris, hyperlipemia, chronic infectious hepatitis, etc.

PHARMACOLOGICAL ACTION 1. Flavonoid glycoside, one of its components, increases coronary flow, reduces myocardial oxygen consumption and lowers arterial pressure.

2. Cardiotonic on frogs' hearts in vitro; low concentration of its extract exerts a vasoconstrictive effect on the vessels of frog's leg and high concentration, vasodilative.

3. Its liquid extract shortens clotting time and exerts hemostatic effect in rabbit.

DIRECTION Powder: 2—5g once or twice daily.

Orientvine Stem
Caulis Sinomenii
Qing feng teng

ORIGIN The vine stem of Sinomenium acutum, family Menispermaceae.

NATURE, TASTE AND CHANNEL TROPISM Acrid and bitter in taste, warm in nature.

EFFICACY AND INDICATION 1. Expel wind-dampness, promote diuresis and alleviate pain: For rheumatism. Recently used for rheumatoid arthritis in which the cellular immunity and immunoglobulin level are found to be normalized. Also for edema and wet beriberi.

2. Lower blood pressure: For hypertension.

PHARMACOLOGICAL ACTION 1. Analgesic, sedative and antitussive.

2. Inhibiting the development of experimental arthritis.

3. Lowering blood pressure rapidly and obviously, but drug tolerance is liable to occur.

DIRECTION Decoction: 9—15g.

This herb may cause side effects such as pruritis, flushing, puffiness of eyelids, allergic purpura, etc.

Peony Root
Radix Paeoniae Rubra
Chi shao

ORIGIN The dried root of Paeonia lactiflora, or several other species of the same genus, family Ranunculaceae.

NATURE, TASTE AND CHANNEL

TROPISM Bitter in taste, slightly cold in nature, and attributive to liver channel.

EFFICACY AND INDICATION 1. Clear away the heat and cool the blood: For seasonal febrile diseases involving xuefen with fever, eruptions and crimson tongue, and blood-heat syndrome with hematemesis or epistaxis.

2. Promote blood circulation to remove blood stasis: For blood-stasis syndrome with amenorrhea, menalgia, chest pain, abdominal pain, abdominal masses, trauma, or skin infection.

3. Clear away liver-fire to promote visual acuity: For liver-heat syndrome with conjunctivitis or hypochondriac pain.

PHARMACOLOGICAL ACTION 1. Paeoniflorin, one of its active components, has a strong antispastic effect and also analgesic, sedative, anticonvulsive, antibacterial and anti-inflammatory effects.

2. Dilating blood vessels, increasing coronary flow and improving myocardial oxygen supply. Hypotensive.

3. Inhibiting platelets aggregation.

DIRECTION Decoction: 6—15g.

Phellodendron Bark
Cortex Phellodendri
Huang bo

ORIGIN The dried bark of Phellodendron chinense or P. amurense, family Rutaceae.

NATURE, TASTE AND CHANNEL TROPISM Bitter in taste, cold in nature, attributive to kidney, urinary bladder and large intestine channels.

EFFICACY AND INDICATION 1. Clear away heat and deprive dampness: For diarrhea, dysentery, jaundice, leucorrhagia, stranguria, etc. of dampness-heat type.

2. Purge the sthenic fire and clear away toxic materials: For skin infection, burn, and seasonal febrile diseases.

3. Purge the kidney-fire and reduce asthenia-heat: For syndrome of fire-hyperactivity and yin-deficiency manifested as hectic fever, night sweat, emission and red-dry tongue.

PHARMACOLOGICAL ACTION Berberine is the main active component with an action similar to Rhizoma Coptidis.

Prepared Rehmannia Root
Radix Rehmanniae Praeparata
Shu di

ORIGIN Root of Rehmannia glutinosa, family Scrophulariaceae.

NATURE, TASTE AND CHANNEL TROPISM Sweet and slightly bitter in tast, slightly warm in nature, acting on heart, liver and kidney channels.

EFFICACY AND INDICATION 1. Produce essence and enrich blood: For insufficiency of essence and blood manifested as sallow complexion, palpitation and menoxenia.

2. Nourish yin and moisturize dryness: For deficiency of liver-yin and kidney-yin manifested as hectic fever, night sweat, emission and diabetes, usually used together with Fructus Corni and Rhizoma Dioscoreae; also used for prurigo due to dryness of blood, muscular spasm due to blood-deficiency or yin-deficiency, and constipation due to insufficiency of body fluid and

blood.

3. Invigorate the liver and kidney: For backache with knee aching due to deficiency of liver and kidney, such as chronic lumbar strain, hyperplasia of lumbar vertebra, etc. Recently used singly for hypertension and hypercholesterinemia.

PHARMACOLOGICAL ACTION 1. Exerting an anti-exudative and anti-inflammatory effect on inflammatory granulation in rats.

2. Cardiotonic hypotensive and diuretic.

3. Catalpol, one of its active components, is an anti-diabetic.

DIRECTION Decoction: 10—30g.

Pueraria Root
Radix Puerariae
Ge gen

ORIGIN The dried root of pueraria lobata, family Leguminosae.

NATURE, TASTE AND CHANNEL TROPISM Sweet and acrid in taste, cool in nature, and attributive to spleen and stomach channels.

EFFICACY AND INDICATION 1. Expel the evil factors from superficies and muscles: For common cold with fever, headache, stiffness and pain of nape and back.

2. Let out the skin eruptions: For measles and measles and macule rash and other eruptive diseases with incomplete eruption, usually used together with Rhizoma Cimicifugae.

3. Lift the lucid yang to ease the upper orifices, and arrest diarrhea: For sudden deafness and blindness (such as central retinitis) due to failure of rising of lucid yang; for diarrhea due to spleen deficiency, used together with Radix Codonopsis Pilosulae, Rhizoma Atractylodis Macrocephalae, etc. ; for diarrhea of dampness-heat type, used together with Rhizoma Coptidis, Radix Scutellariae, etc.

4. Promote the production of body fluid to quench thirst: For superficial heat-syndrome with thirst, febrile disease with body fluid consumption, spleen deficiency with thirst, and diabetes. Recently, used for hemicrania, stiff neck, hypertensive headache, neck pain, tinnitus and coronary heart disease.

PHARMACOLOGICAL ACTION 1. Its active component, daidzein, can dilate the coronary and cerebral arteries.

2. Its decoction and extract are mild hypotensives.

3. Oral administration of its extractum reduces vaccine-induced fever in rabbits.

4. Antispastic.

DIRECTION Decoction: 6—20g.

Radish Seed
Semen Raphani
Lai fu zi

ORIGIN Seed of Raphanus sativus, family Cruciferae.

NATURE, TASTE AND CHANNEL TROPISM Acrid and sweet in taste, mild in nature, and attributive to lung, spleen and stomach channels.

EFFICACY AND INDICATION 1. Promote digestion and relieve dyspepsia: For serious cases of dyspepsia with chest upset, abdominal distension, eructation, acid regurgitation, constipation, or diarrhea; for habitual constipation, single use or mixed with honey.

2. Eliminate phlegm and descend the adverse-rising energy: For productive cough and dyspnea.

3. Lower blood pressure: For hypertension.

PHARMACOLOGICAL ACTION 1. Raphanin, one of its active components, inhibits the growth of Staphylococcus and Bacillus coli in vitro.

2. Intravenous injection of its aqueous extract exerts hypotensive effect in anesthetized rabbits.

3. Anti-inflammatory.

DIRECTION Decoction: 6 — 12g, 15 — 30g for constipation of sthenia-syndrome; 50-70g for hypertension.

Powder: 9-12g for habitual constipation.

Red Ochre
Ochra Haematitum
Dai zhe shi

ORIGIN This drug is the ore of Hematite(trigonal system).

NATURE, TASTE AND CHANNEL TROPISM Bitter in taste, cold in nature, acting on liver and heart channels.

EFFICACY AND INDICATION   1. Calming the liver and suppressing hyperactivity of the liver-yang, checking and desending the upward adverse flow of qi, removing heat from the blood and stopping bleeding.

2. For headache and dizziness due to hyperactivity of the liver-yang.

3. Eructation, hiccup, vomiting and dyspnea: For eructation and vomiting due to deficiency of the stomach and retention of phlegm; for the relief of reversed upward flow of qi and asthma due to deficiency of both the lung and kidney, it can be used with dangshen and dogwood fruit.

4. Bleeding due to invasion of heat into the blood: Such as hematemesis and epistaxis.

DIRECTION Decoction: 10—30g, decocted first. For checking the upward adverse flow of qi and calming the liver, it is used unprepared for arresting bleeding, preferably calcined. This drug shoule be used cautiously for women in pregnancy.

Rhubarb
Radix et Rhizoma Rhei
Da huang

ORIGIN The root and rhizome of Rheum palmatum, R. tanguticum or R. officinale, family Polygonaceae.

NATURE, TASTE AND CHANNEL TROPISM Bitter in taste, cold in nature, and attributive to spleen, stomach, large intestine, liver and pericardium channels.

EFFICACY AND INICATION 1. Promote digestion and relieve dyspepsia, purge heat and clear away toxic materials: (1) For constipation of sthenia-heat type with coma, delirium, convulsion, mania or abdominal distension and pain (Decoction for potent purgation); (2) For syndrome resulting from evils accumulating in the thorax with abdominal distension and pain, tenderness, dry tongue and thirst, hectic fever, or shortness of breath and listlessness (Decoction for severe phlegm-heat syndrome in the chest); (3) For acute appendicitis; (4) For dysentery of dampness-heat type with abdominal pain and tenesmus; (5) Single use for biliary infection, cholelithiasis and pancreatitis; for biliary ascariasis; (6) For acute and simple intestinal obstruction, roundworm intestinal obstruction and paralytic intestinal obstruction, Decoction for potent purgation may be used; (7) For food and drug poisoning; (8) For pulmonary heart disease with respiratory failure and constipation; (9) For cold-syndrome with constipation, used together with aconite root, dried ginger.

2. Clear away heat and toxic materials: Oral and external use for furuncle and carbuncle due to intense heat; topical use for burn of medirm or small size, cervical erosion and mycotic vaginitis; also for sorethroat, conjunctival congestion, aphthae and toothache due to domination of fire.

3. Stop bleeding: For peptic ulcer with bleeding, also for hemoptysis and epistaxis due to blood stasis, blood-heat or domination of fire.

4. Promote blood circulation and remove blood stasis: For trauma, especially those of the chest and abdomen with constipation; amenia, dysmenorrhea and postpartum abdominal pain due to blood stasis.

5. Chologogue and relieve jaundice: For preventing and treating icterus neonatorum, used together

with Herba Artemisiae Scopariae, Radix Scutellariae, Radix Glycyrrhizae; for icteric viral jaundice, and acute and serious cases of hepatitis.

PHARMACOLOGICAL ACTION 1. Sennoside A is the main component for purgation.

2. Promoting biliary secretion and enhancing the amount of bilirubin and bile acid.

3. Rhein and Emodin exert bacteriostatic effect by inhibiting the synthesis of DAN, RNA and protein in bacteria.

4. Emodin is a component for hypotensive.

5. Chrysophanol, another active component, exerts a hemostatic effect.

DIRECTION Decoction: 3 — 12g. Powder: 2 — 5g, daily dose 4 — 10g. For purgation, decoct later (only boil for 15 minutes)or soak in the boiled water for oral use.

Root-bark of Chinese Wolfberry
Cortex Lycii Radicis
Di gu pi

ORIGIN The root bark of Lycium chinensis and L. barbarum, family Solanaceae.

NATURE, TASTE AND CHANNEL TROPISM   Bitter and bland in taste, cold in nature, and attributive to lung and kidney channels.

EFFICACY AND INDICATION 1. Lower asthenic fever: For fever due to yin-deficiency and the late stage of febrile disease with yin-consumption, manifested as fever high at night and subsided in the morning, hectic fever, night sweat, red and dry tongue without fur, etc, and for infantile malnutrition with fever, usually used together with Rhizoma Anemarrhenae, Carapax Trionycis, etc.

2. Clear away heat and cool the blood: For hematemesis, epistaxis, hemoptysis and hematuria due to blood-heat.

3. Clear away lung-heat: For cough and dyspnea due to lung-heat, usually used together with Cortex Mori Radicis, Radix Gylycyrrhizae, Fructus oryzae

Sativae(Powder for expelling lung-heat).

4. Lower blood pressure: For hypertension. In addition, also for tuberculous lymphadenitis, urticaria, allergic purpura, drug rash, allergy to insect bite, etc.

PHARMACOLOGICAL ACTION 1. Its decoction, infusion, tincture and injection exert a hypotensive effect on anesthetized or unanesthetized animals.

2. Antipyretyic. Reducing vaccine-induced fever in rabbits.

3. Its extract lowers serum cholesterol level in rabbits.

4. Its decoction reduces blood sugar level in rabbits.

5. An active component, betaine, possesses a lipocaic effect.

DIRECTION Decoction: 6—12g.

Root-bark of White Mulberry
Cortex Mori Radicis
Sang bai pi

ORIGIN The root epidermis of Morus alba, family Moraceae.

NATURE, TASTE AND CHANNEL TROPISM Sweet in teste, cold in nature, and attributive to lung channel.

EFFICACY AND INDICATION 1. Purge lung-fire, eliminate phlegm and relieve dyspnea: For lung-heat syndrome with productive cough and dyspnea, usually used together with Cortex Lycii Radicis, Radix Glycyrrhizae and Fructus Oryzae Sativae; for fluid-retention syndrome involving the lung manifested as distension of the chest, cough with thin sputum, dyspnea and edema of face, used together with Herba Ephedrae, Semen Armeniacae Amarum and herba Asari.

2. Promote diuresis and reduce edema: For edema and dysuria.

3. Lower blood pressure: For hypertension.

PHARMACOLOGICAL ACTION Its extract is hypotensive, cardio-inhibitory and vasoconstrictive, and excites the intestines and uterus in experimental animals.

DIRECTION Decoction: 9—18g.

Root of Fourstamen Stephania
Radix Stephaniae Tetrandrae
Fen fang ji

ORIGIN Root of Stephania tetrandra, family Menispermaceae.

NATURE, TASTE AND CHANNEL TROPISM   Bitter in taste, cold in nature, and attributive to lung, spleen and urinary bladder channels.

EFFICACY AND INDICATION   1. Expel wind-dampness and alleviate pain: For arthralgia, especially of heat type, also for acrodynia of dampness-heat type, trauma, periarthritis of joint and angina pectoris.

2. Promote diuresis and relieve edema: For edema and dysuria.

3. Eliminate phlegm and relieve asthma: In ancient times, use for dyspneic cough due to "withered " lung or lung-heat; for hemoptysis with abundant expectoration due to withered lung, used together with Semen Lepidii seu Descurainiae. Recently, used for bronchial asthma, asthmatic bronchitis, silicosis, pulmonary tuberculosis, etc.

4. Lower blood pressure: For hypertension, especially that complicated by coronary heart diseases.

5. Anti-carcinogenic: For carcinoma of lung, and squamous cell epithioma (decreasing the dosage of radiotherapy by one-third to one-fourth and minimizing the occurrence of side effect).

PHARMACOLOGICAL ACTION 1. Hanfangchin A and B are two active components, which have an anti-inflammatory effect.

2. Anti-allergic, inhibiting the release of histamine.

3. Promoting phagocytosis.

4. Dilating coronary artery and decreasing myocardial oxygen cosumption.

5. Inhibiting the growth of Bacillus tuberculosis, Staphylococcus aureus and ameba.

6. High dosage may induce respiratory inhibition and cardiac arrest.

DIRECTION Decoction: 6—12g.

Table (Hanfangchin A 20 or 60mg): tid.; or 200 —300 mg tid. for tumor.

Ampoule (Hanfangchin A 60mg): 120 mg added in normal saline 20 ml IV daily, or 30—60mg IM bid.

Tetrandrine, an effective alkaloid extracted from

Radix Stephaniae Tetrandrae, can be given intravenously for severe hypertension or malignant hypertension at a dose of 120—180mg. It can also be administered orally in long-term treatment of primary hypertension at a doee of 100mg, three times a day. Its effective rate is 69 percent, yet is does not cause postural hypotension or other side effects, or impair the liver and kidneys.

Root of Pubescent Holly
Radix Ilicis Pubescentis
Mao dong qing

ORIGIN The root of Ilex pubescens, family Aquifoliaceae.

NATURE, TASTE AND CHANNEL TROPISM Bitter in taste, cold in nature, and attributive to heart and lung channels.

EFFICACY AND INDICATION 1. Promote blood circulation to remove blood stasis, dredge the channels and collaterals: For blood stasis syndrome with angina pectoris, ischemic apoplexy, thromboantiitis obliterans, arteritis, central retinitis, uveitis, hypertension, hypercholesterinemia, etc.

2. Clear away heat and toxic materials: For skin infection, burn, wound infection, etc., both for oral and ex ernal use.

3. Eliminate phlegm, and relieve cough and asthma: For lung-heat syndrome with cough and asthma.

PHARMACOLOGICAL ACTION 1. Dilating the coronary artery and increasing coronary flow for rabbit's heart in vitro and dog's heart in vivo.

2. Exerting slow and sustained hypotensive effect in anesthetized cats or dogs.

3. Antitussive and expectorant.

DIRECTION Decoction: 30 — 60g, up to 60 — 150g as necessary. Injection: Injectio Ilicis Pubescentis 2 — 4 ml IM 2 — 4 times daily; Injectio Ilicin A 20mg added in glucose solution IV in drips for ischemic apoplexy. Tablet (containing 100mg of extract): 3 — 4 tablets tid.

Safflower
Flos Carthami
Hong hua

ORIGIN The flower of Carthamus tinctorius, family Compositae.

NATURE,TASTE AND CHANNEL TROPISM
Acrid in taste, warm in nature, and attributive to heart and liver channels.

EFFICACY AND INDICATION 1. Promote blood circulation to remove blood stasis, promote menstruation and alleviate pain: For blood-stasis syndrome with amenia, dysmenorrhea, or postpartum abdominal pain. Recently, for ischemic apoplexy, angina pectoris, thromboangiitis obliterans, sudden deafness, sclerederma neonatorum,flat wart, neurodermatitis,etc.

2. Promote blood circulation to relieve carbuncle: For preventing and treating bed sore (external use); for conjunctivitis and the early stage of the carbuncle.

3. Promote blood circulation and let out the skin eruption: For blood stasis with impediment of skin eruptions.

PHARMACOLOGICAL ACTION 1. Its decoc-

216

tion stimulates uteri and intestines of experimental animals in vitro.

2. Its decoction increases coronary flow and lowers blood pressure in dogs.

3. Small dose of its decoction mildly stimulates and large dose inhibits the heart of toads.

DIRECTION Decoction: 0. 6 — 1. 0g for promoting blood production; 2. 0 — 2. 5g for regulating blood; 3 — 9g promoting blood circulation; 9 — 12g for removing blood stasis.

Injection: 50% solution 2 — 4 ml IM once or twice daily; for ischemic apolexy, 10 — 15 ml added in 10% glucose injection 250 ml IV for drips daily, 15 — 20 times as 1 course.

Scorpion
Scorpio
Quan xie

ORIGIN The whole body of Buthus martensii, family Buthidae.

NATURE, TASTE AND CHANNEL TROPISM Sweet and acrid in taste, mild in nature, toxic, and attributive to liver channel.

EFFICACY AND INDICATION 1. Expel wind and relieve spasm: For tetanus, acute and chronic infantile convulsion. apoplexy, with distortion of the face.

2. Dredge the meridian and alleviate pain: For headache of head-wind or blood-stasis type, rheumatism, etc.

3. Remove toxic material and disperse the lumps: For skin infection, scrofula and subcutaneous nodes.

PHARMACOLOGICAL ACTION 1. Anti-convulsive and sedative.

2. Exerting significant and prolonged hypotensive effect.

3. Buthotoxin can induce respiratory paralysis, salivation and convulsion.

DIRECTION   Decoction: 2—5g. Powder: 0. 6 —1. 0 g bid or tid.

Scutellaria Root
Radix Scutellariae
Huang qin

ORIGIN The dried root of scutellaria baicalensis, family Labiatae.

NATURE, TASTE AND CHANNEL TROPISM Bitter in taste, cold in nature, and attributive to lung, gallbladder and large intestine channels.

EFFICACY AND INDICATION 1. Clear away heat and deprive dampness from the middle-jiao: For diarrhea, dysentery and jaundice of dampness type, dampness-heat diseases in summer, stranguria of heat tupe. Recently, also used for acute biliary infection.

2. Purge the sthenic fire and detoxify: For dyspneic cough due to lung-heat, pharyngitis, and seasonal febrile disease. Recently baicalin is used for epidemic B encephalitis.

3. Purge the sthenic fire to stop bleeding: For heat-syndrome with hematemesis, hemoptysis, hemafecia or epistaxis.

4. Lower the blood pressure: For hypertension, especially those with flushed face listlessness and red

tongue with yellow coating.

PHARMACOLOGICAL ACTION 1. Possessing a broad-spectrum bacteriostatic and virustatic effect.

2. Anti-allergic and anti-inflammatory.

3. Intravenous injection or oral administration of its decoction can lower typhoid vaccine-induced fever in rabbits.

4. Hypotensive.

5. Acting as a cholcogogue and relaxing the spasms of small intestine.

DIRECTION Decoction: 3—9g.

Tablet (containing baicalin 250 mg): 2—3 tablets tid.

Ampoule (containing baicalin 60mg in 2ml): 1—2 ampoules IM 1—2 times daily, or 8—20ml in 10% glucose injection 500ml IV for drips daily.

Sophora Flower
Flos Sophorae
Huai hua

ORIGIN The flower bud of Sophora japonica, family Leguminosae.

NATURE, TASTE AND CHANNEL TROPISM Bitter in taste, mild in nature, and attributive to stomach, liver and large intestine channels.

EFFICACY AND INDICATION 1. Cool the blood and stop bleeding: Generally used for hemorrhoids, hematemesis and hemafecia, also for hemoptysis, metrorrhagia, etc.

2. Clear away liver-heat and lower blood pressure: For hypertension.

PHARMACOLOGICAL ACTION 1. Its component rutin decreases capillary permeability.

2. Lowering blood pressure transiently in anesthetized dog.

3. Inhibiting the growth of various dermatomyces.

DIRECTION Decoction: 9—12g up to 30—60g.

Tend Twig and Leaf of
Harlequin Glorybower
Ramulus et Folium Clerodendri Trichotomi
Chou wu tong

ORIGIN The dried tender twig and leaf of Clerodendrum trichotomum, family Verbenaceae.

NATURE, TASTE AND CHANNEL TROPISM Bitter and sweet in taste, cold in nature, and attributive to liver, gallbladder and lung channels.

EFFICACY AND INDICATION 1. Expel wind-dampness and relieve pain: For rheumatism, apoplexy complicated by hemiplegia, and migraine; also for prurigo of dampness-heat type and carbuncle.

2. Lower blood pressure: For hypetension, used singly or together with Lumbricus.

3. Antimalarial.

4. Eliminate sputum, relieve cough and dyspnea: For chronic bronchitis.

PHARMACOLOGICAL ACTION Clerodendronin A and B are the chief active components.

1. Oral administration or intramuscular injection of its decoction exerts a hypotensive effect which may be attributable to the dilatation of blood vessels and the blockage of vegetative ganglia.

2. Combined use of this drug and Herba Siegesbeckiae is inhibitory on the experimental arthritis, but no such effect is observed when they are used individually.

3. Clerodendronin A or B is a sedative and anal-

gesic respectively.

DIRECTION Decoction: 10—15g.

Tablet (containing clerodendronin A 30mg): 30mg bid or tid for hypertension, followed by 30—60mg qd after the blood pressure becomes normal.

Uncaria Stem with Hooks
Ramulus Uncariae cum Uncis
Gou teng

ORIGIN The hooked vine of Uncaria rhynchopylla, U. macrophylla, and U. hirsuta, family Rubiaceae.

NATURE, TASTE AND CHANNEL TROPISM Sweet in taste, slightly cold in nature, and attributive to liver, heart and pericardium channels.

EFFICACY AND INDICATION 1. Clear away and calm the liver, expel wind and relieve spasm: For heat syndrome with convulsion, especially infantile convulsion; for hyperactivity or wind-transformation of liver-yang with dizziness, headache, listlessness, and numbness, tremor and spasm of extremities; for aerious liver-fire syndrome manifested as epilepsy and insanity, used together with Lumbricus and Cornu

Saigae Tataricae.

2. Clear away liver-fire and improve visual acuity: For liver-heat syndrome with conjunctivitis and headache.

3. Expel wind clear away heat: For wind-heat affection with fever, headache and conjunctival congestion, prurigo of wind-heat type.

4. Lower blood pressure: For hypertension, especially that attributive to hyperactivity of liver-yang.

PHARMACOLOGICAL ACTION 1. Its decoction lowers blood pressure in anesthetized or unanesthetized animals. The active component is Rhynchophylline.

2. Intraperitoneal injection of its decoction exerts sedative effect in mice.

3. Hypodermic injection of its alcoholic infusion exerts an antiepileptic effect in guinea-pigs.

4. Antispasmodic.

DIRECTION Decoction: 10 — 15g (decocted later). It is indicated for treatment of mind and moderate hypertension.

White Peony Root
Radix Paeoniae Alba
Bai shao

ORIGIN Root of Paeonia lactiflora, family Ranunculaceae.

NATURE, TASTE AND CHANNEL TROPISM Bitter and sour in taste, slightly cold in nature, and acting on liver channel.

EFFICACY AND INDICATION 1. Nourish blood and astringe yin: For yin-deficiency and blood-deficiency manifested as menoxenia, menalgia, leucorrhagia and metrorrhagia, usually used together with Radix Rehmanniae and Radix Angelicae Sinensis; for night sweat due to yin-deficiency and spontaneous perspiration due to low body resistance and imbalance between ying-energy and wei-energy, used together with Ramulus Cinnamomi; for muscular spasm and pain of extremities due to blood deficiency, usually used together with Radix Glycyrrhizae; for rheumatism due to insufficiency of yin-blood.

2. Calm liver yang: For deficiency of yin leading to hyperactivity of yang and sthenia of liver-yang mani-

fested as dizziness, headache, irritability and insomnia; also for convulsion of wind-syndrome resulting from sthenic liver-yang, severe heat, yin-deficiency or blood-deficiency.

3. Soothe the liver and alleviate pain: For abnormal rising of liver energy or dominant liver energy attacking stomach manifested as pain in the chest and abdomen.

PHARMACOLOGICAL ACTION 1. Dilating the coronary artery and blood vessels of hind legs in dogs.

2. Lowering blood pressure transiently.

3. Inhibiting the intestines in rabbits in vitro.

4. Its component paeoniflorin inhibits the central nervous system.

DIRECTION Decoction: 6—15g.

Wild Jujube Seed
Semen Ziziphi Spinosae
Suan zao ren

ORIGIN Seed of Ziziphus spinosa, family Rhamnaceae.

NATURE, TASTE AND CHANNEL TROPISM Sweet and sour in taste, mind in nature, and attributive to heart and liver channels.

EFFICACY AND INDICATION 1. Nourish the heart, benefit the liver and tranquilize the mind: For deficiency of heart-blood and liver-blood with vexation, insomnia, severe palpitation, frightening and amnesia, used together with Radix Angelicae Sinensis, Radix Polygoni Multiflori and Arillus Longan; for liver-deficiency with heat, used together with Rhizoma Anemarrhenae and Poria; for yin-deficiency with yang-hyperactivity, used together with Radix Rehmanniae and Semen Biotae.

2. Stop sweating: For general debility with spontaneous perspiration, and night sweating.

PHARMACOLOGICAL ACTION The chief components are jujuboside A and B.

1. Intraperitoneal injection of its decoction(2.5 — 5.0g/kg) exerts sedative and hypnotic effects in rats.

2. Intravenous injection of its decoction exerts significant and prolonged hypotensive effect in anesthetized dogs.

3. Occasionally causing heart block.

4. Inducing hysterospasm.

DIRECTION Decoction: 9—18g.

Results from experiment studies in animal models of hypertension showed that the following traditional Chinese medicines have antihypertensive action: Dutchmanspipe root (Radix Aristolochiae), Herb of Black Nightshade (Herba Solani Nigri), Cucumber stem (Caulis cucumeris sativi), Fruit of Chinese Azale (Fructus Rhododendri Mollis) etc.

Chapter Four
PRESCRIPTIONS OF TCM
FOR LOWERING BLOOD PRESSURE

Antidotal Decoction of Coptis
(Huang lian jie du tang)

INGREDIENTS

Rhizoma Coptidis 9g

Radix Scutellariae 6g

Cortex Phellodendri 6g

Fructus Gardeniae 9g

EFFICACY AND INDICATIONS   Purging pathogenic fire and lessening virulence of any pathogenic organism.

All the syndromes of fire-toxin by excessive heat or intense heat in the tri-warmer manifested by high fever, fidgetiness, dry mouth and lips, dysentery with fever, jaundice due to damp-heat, reddened tongue with yellow coating, and rapid and forceful pulse.

The recipe can also be modified to treat many other disorders. For example, influenza, encephalitis B, epidemic cerebrospinal meningitis, septicemia, acute infectious hepatitis, bacillary dysentery and others that belong to syndromes of fire-toxin and excessive heat, disorder of vegetative nervous function, hypertension, which indicate the syndrome of intense heat in the heart and stomach or excessive fire in the liver and gall-bladder.

INTERPRETATION In the recipe, coptis root is used as a principal drug which plays a significant role in purging pathogenic fire in the heart and stomach. Scutellaria root acts as an assistant drug with the effect of clearing away heat in the lung and purging fire in the upper-warmer. No. 3 and No. 4, cortex phellodendri and Fructus Gardeniae, are used in combination as both adjuvant and guiding drugs, the former providing the effect of purging pathogenic fire in the lower-warmer and the latter having the effect of removing pathogenic fire in the tri-warmer by inducing diuresis. The combination of the four ingredients results in the disappearance of both fire-pathogen and heat-toxin. The health condition thus becomes normal.

Modern researches have confirmed that the recipe can exert the function of relieving inflammation, allaying fever, resisting bacteria and viruses, and tranquiliz-

230

ing the mind. In addition, it has the virtue to normalize the function of the gallbladder, arrest bleeding, promote diuresis, and reduce blood pressure.

CAUTIONS The recipe is fit for cases with overabundance of heat-toxin in the tri-warmer but no impairment of the body fluid. So it is not advisable for those with injury of the body fluid by heat manifested as deep-red and uncoated tongue.

Antihypertensive Tablet
(Jiang ya ping pian)

INGREDIENTS
Prunella spike (Spica prunellae)
Scutellaria root (Radix Scutellariae)
Mother of pearl (Concha Margaritifera Usta)
Chrysanthemum flower (Flos Chrysanthemi)
Mistletoe (Herba Visci)
Earthworm (Lumbricus)
Peppermint (Herba Menthae)
Tablets, 0.3g each tablet, 12 tablets per vial, 10 vials per box.

EFFICACY Relieving hypertension and refreshing

oneself.

INDICATIONS Hypertension and dizziness.

DIRECTION To be taken orally, 4 tablets each time, 3 times a day.

Bolus as Kidney-yin-tonic
(Zuo gui wan)

INGREDIENTS

Rhizoma Rehmanniae Praeparata 240g

    Rhizoma Dioscoreae 120g

    Fructus Lycii 120g

    Fructus Corni 120g

    Radix Cyathulae 90g

    Semen Cuscutae 120g

    Colla Cornus Cervi 120g

    Colla Plastri Testudinis 120g

EFFICACY AND INDICATIONS Nourishing yin and tonifying the kidney. Syndrome of deficiency of genuine yin marked by vertigo, lassitude in the loins and legs, seminal emission or spermatorrhea, spontaneous perspiration, night sweat, dry mouth and throat, thirst with desire for drinks, smooth tongue with little coating, and thready or rapid pulse.

Besides, syndrome of deficiency of genuine yin occurring in cases of debilitated constitution due to advanced age, chronic disorders, or recovery stage of febrile diseases can be treated with the modified recipe.

INTERPRETATION In the recipe, Prepared rhizome of rehmannia, great in dosage, is used to nourish the kidney-yin; No. 3, Wolfberry fruit is to supplement the essence of life and improve acuity of vision; and No. 4, Dogwood fruit is to astringe seminal emission and sweating. Both No. 7 Antler glue and No. 8 Tortoise-plastron glue, which have close relation to health, are used in combination for replenishing and tonifying the essence, with the former tending to tonify yang and the latter tending to nourish yin. No. 6, Dodder Seed assisted by Cyathula root, has the effect of strengthening the waist and knees and reinforcing the muscles and joints. No. 2 Chinese yam gives the effect of nourishing and replenishing the spleen and kidney.

DIRECTIONS The boluses are made out of the powdered drugs with honey. Each bolus weighs 9g. One bolus is to be taken each time with slightly salty liquid in the early morning and before bed time on an empty stomach.

Bolus for Serious
Endogenous wind-Syndrome
（Da ding feng zhu）

INGREDIENTS
Radix Paeoniae Alba 18g
Radix Rehmanniae 18g
Colla Corii Asini 10g
Radix Ophiopogonis 10g
Plastrum Testudinis(decocted first)12g
Concha Ostreae(decocted first)12g
Carapax Trionycis(decocted first)12g
Semen Sesami 6g
Fructus Schisandrae 6g
Fresh Egg Yolk(mixed with decoction)1
Radix Glycyrrhizae Praeparata 3g

EFFICACY Nourishing yin and calming wind; mainly for cases of clonic convulsion attributive to damage of true-yin by heat and hyperactivity of liver-wind, which are accompanied with listlessness, crimson and uncoated tongue, small and weak pulse.

INDICATIONS 1. Indicated for cases attributive

to deficiency of liver-yin and kidney-yin and upward attack of liver-yang, which are manifested as dizziness aggravated by over strain or angry, soreness of the loins and knees, sleeplessness, dreamfulness, nocturnal emission, fatigue, bright red tongue, small and rapid pulse.

2. Also applicable to cases of encephalitis B, epidemic meningitis, poliomyelitis and chorea, marked by convulsion, which are attributive to damage of true-yin by heat and hyperactivity of liver-wind.

3. Also applicable to case of hypertension, which is manifested as hyperactivity of liver-wind.

INTERPRETATION Egg yolk and colla Corii Asini are applied to nourish yin-fluid, supplement the exhausted true-yin and calm liver-wind. Rehmanniae, Sesami, Ophiopogonis and Paeoniae Alba serve to nourish yin and blood, soothe the liver and calm wind. Plastrum Testudinis, Concha Ostreae and Carapax Trionycis can invigorate kidney-yin and suppress the hyperactive liver-yang. Glycyrrhizae Praeparata and Schisandrae are helpful for yin nourishing and wind calming.

Bolus for Tonifying
the Kidney-qi
(Shen qi wan).

INGREDIENTS

Radix Rehmanniae 240g

Rhizoma Dioscoreae 120g

Fructus Corni 120g

Rhizoma Alismatis 90g

Poria 90g

Cortex Moutan Radicis 90g

Ramulus Cinnamomi 30g

Radix Aconiti Praeparata (stir-baked at high temperature) 30g

EFFICACY AND INDICATIONS Warming and tonifying the kidney-yang. Insufficiency of the kidney-yang manifested by lassitude in the loins, legs and feet, cold feeling in the lower part of the body, stiffness in the lower abdomen, dysphoria with smothery sensation resulting in inability to lie flat but rest against bed instead, dysuria or polyuria, bulgy and pale tongue, feeble pulse or deep and faint pulse.

Equally, the above syndrome occurring in chronic

nephritis, diabetes, vegetative nerve disturbance, senile dementia, and other chronic disorders, or urinary dysfunction may be treated with the modified recipe.

DIRECTIONS One bolus is to be taken in the morning and another in the evening with warm boiled water. Or instead, the drugs are decocted proportionately with reference to the dosage of the original recipe.

INTERPRETATION Of all the ingredients in the recipe, the first three are all used as tonics, the first replenishing the kidney-yin while the second and the third nourishing the liver and spleen to reinforce the effect of the first one. The last two drugs which are dosed the least are used to warm and replenish the kidney-yang. No. 4 and No. 5, Rhizoma Alismatis and Poria play their part in removing dampness and promoting diuresis. No. 6, Cortex Moutan Radicis, has the effect of removing liver-fire and is coordinated with the invigorators for kidney-yang to produce the consequence of coexistance of both invigorating and purging action for the purpose of getting rid of the greasy side effect involved in the invigorating action.

Modern researches have proved that this recipe has the efficacies in improving hypophysis-adrenocortical function, promoting blood circulation, tranquilizing the mind, lowering blood pressure, strengthening kidney function, protecting the liver and so on.

CAUTIONS It is not advisable to administer this recipe for patients with hyperactivity of fire due to yin deficiency and impairment of body fluid due to dryness-heat.

Bolus of Cinnamomi and Poria
(Gui zhi fu ling wan)

INGREDIENTS
Ramulus Cinnamomi 10g
Cortex Moutan Radicis 10g
Poria 15g
Semen Persicae 6g
Radix Paeoniae Rubra 12g
Prepared with honey into boluses.

EFFICACY Activating blood circulation, removing blood stasis and abdominal mass; mainly for cases attributive to the blending of phlegm and blood stasis, which are manifested as tender masses in the lower abdomen and unsmooth pulse.

INDICATIONS 1. For cases of irregular menstruation，amenorrhea，retention of the dead fetus，lochiostasis，etc.，which are attributive to the accumulation of blood stasis and phlegm in the lower jiao.

2. Also applicable to cases of hysteromyoma，metropolypus，ovarian cyst，salpingitis，pelvic cellulitis，etc.，marked by pain or masses over the lower abdomen，which are attributive to the accumulation of blood stasis and phlegm.

3. Also applicable to arteriosclerosis，hypentension，etc.，which are attributive to the accumulation of blood stasis.

INTERPRETATION Ramulus Cinnamomi here is not used for expelling the superficies evils from the body surface as usual; it acts with Persicae，Paeoniae Rubra and Moutan Radicis to activate blood circulation and eliminate blood stasis and abdominal mass. Poria acts with Ramulus Cinnamomi to disperse phlegm and dampness evil which are considered as other causes of abdominal masses.

DIRECTION To be taken orally，A. C.，with warm boiled water，1 boluse each time，or 2 boluses for serious Cases，three times a day.

Bolus of Cow-bezoar for
Clearing Heart-fire
(Wan shi niu huang qing xin wan)

INGREDIENTS
Cow-bezoar (Calculus Bovis)
Curcuma (Radix Curcumae)
Capejasmine (Fructus Gardeniae)
Coptis root (Rhizoma coptidis)
Cinnabar (Cinnabaris)
Scutellaria root (Radix Scutellariae)
Honeyed boluses, 3g each bolus, 10 boluses per box.

EFFICACY Removing heat from the heart to restore consciousness and reducing heat and eliminating phlegm for resuscitation.

INDICATIONS The accumulation of heat-phlegm in the body, and the attack of pericardium by heat, manifested as stroke, coma, delirium, listlessness, wheezing sound and abundant expectoration, high fever and convulsion.

DIRECTION To be taken orally, with warm boiled water, 1 — 2 boluses each time, twice a day.

Children: the doses should be reduced correspondingly.

Never administered to patients with deficiency syndrome.

Bolus of Gentian for Purging Liver-fire
(Long dan xie gan wan)

INGREDIENTS

Gentian root (Radix Gentianae)

Bupleurum root (Radix Bupleuri)

Scutellaria root (Radix Scutellariae)

Capejasmine fruit (Fructus Gardeniae)

Oriental water plantain rhizome (Rhizoma Alismatis)

Akebia stem (Caulis Akebiae)

Plantain seed (Semen Plantaginis)

Chinese Angelica root (Radix Angelicae Sinensis)

Rehmannia root (Radix Rehmanniae)

Liquorice (Radix Glycyrrhizae)

Grind the above drugs into fine powder, mix it with honey and make them into bolus, 9g each bolus, 10 boluses per box.

EFFICACY Clearing away pathogenic fire in the liver and gallbladder, removing dampness and heat.

INDICATIONS Fire of excess type or dampness-heat in the liver and gallbladder manifested as dizziness, conjunctival congestion, otalgia, tinnitus, hypochondriac pain, bitter taste, dark urine, difficulty and pain in micturition.

DIRECTION To be taken orally, 9g each time, twice a day.

It should be given to pregnant women with great care.

Bolus of Six Drugs
Including Rehmannia
(Liu wei di huang wan)

INGREDIENTS

Rhizoma Rehmanniae Praeparata 240g

Fructus Corni 120g

Rhizoma Dioscoreae 120g

Rhizoma Alismatis 90g

Poria 90g

Cortex Moutan Radicis 90g

Grind the above drugs into fine powder and mix

with honey to make boluses, to be administered orally 6 — 9 grams each time with warm boiled water, 2 — 3 times a day.

EFFICACY Nourishing and enriching the liver and kidney.

INDICATIONS Syndrome due to the deficiency of vital essence of liver and kidney with symptoms of weakness and soreness of waist and knees, vertigo, deafness, night sweat, emission as well as persistant opening of fontanel. Or the flaring up of sthenic fire resulting in symptoms such as hectic fever, feverish sensation in the palms and soles, diabetes or toothache due to fire of deficiency type, dry mouth and throat, red tongue with little fur, and thready and rapid pulse.

In addition, the above recipe can be modified to treat many other disease indicating the syndrome due to the deficiency of vital essence of liver and kidney such as vegetative nerve functional disturbance, hypertension, arteriosclerosis, diabets, chronic nephritis, hyperthyroidism, pulmonary tuberculosis, chronic urinary infection, bronchial asthma, amenorrhea, scanty menstruation, or infantile dysplasis and interlectual hypoevolutism.

INTERPRETATION Prepared rhizome of

rehmannia, as the principal one, possesses the effect of nourishing the kidney-yin and supplementing the essence of life. As assistant drugs, Dogwood fruit, sour in flavor and warm in nature, is used for nourishing the kidney and replenishing the liver, while Dried Chinese yam for nourishing the kidney-yin and tonifying the spleen. The rest ingredients collectively play the role of adjuvant drugs. Oriental water plantain coordinates with the principal drug in clearing the kidney and purging turbid evils, Cortex Moutan Radicis cooperates with Dogwood fruit in purging liver fire, and Poria shares the effort together with Dried Chinese yam to excrete dampness from the spleen. The whole recipe acts as both tonics and purgatives with tonifying effect dominant.

Clinically and experimentally, the recipe has the effects of nourishing the body and consolidating the constitution, inhibiting hypercatabolism, reducing excitement of the brain, adjusting endocrine function and vegetative nerve, lowering blood pressure and blood sugar, inducing diuresis, improving the function of the kidney as well as promoting the epithelial hyperplasia of the esophagus and preventing cancer, etc.

CAUTIONS Since it tends to be greasy tonics,

the recipe should be administered carefully to patients with weakened function of the spleen in transporting and distributing nutrients and water.

Cardiotonic Pill
(Tian wang bu xin dan)

INGREDIENTS

Radix Rehmanniae 120g

Radix Scrophulariae 60g

Radix Salviae Miltiorrhizae 60g

Radix Angelicae Sinensis 60g

Radix Ginseng 60g

Poria 60g

Semen Biotae 60g

Semen Ziziphi Spinosae 60g

Radix Polygalae 60g

Radix Asparagi 60g

Radix Ophiogonis 60g

Fructus Schisandrae 60g

Radix Platycodi 60g

Take 9 grams three times a day. It can also be made into decoction, with the dosage modified proportionally according to the original recipe.

EFFICACY AND INDICATIONS Nourishing yin to remove heat and tonifying the blood to tranquilize the mind. Deficiency-fire stirring up inside due to deficiency of yin and blood brought on by the hypofunction of heart and kidney marked by insomnia with vexation, palpitation, mental weariness, nocturnal emission, amnesia, dry stools, orolingual boil, reddened tongue with little fur, thready and rapid pulse.

Neurosism, paroxysmal tachycardia, hy)ertension, hyperthyroidism and others marked by the above-mentioned symptoms can be treated by the modified recipe.

Modern researches have proved that the recipe has a better effect of regulating the cerbral cortex. It can tranquilize the mind to induce sleep without causing listlessness and achieve the effects of enriching the blood and relieving the symptoms of coronary heart disease.

CAUTIONS The recipe is composed of nourishing, greasy drugs which affect the stomach, so it is not fit to take for a long time.

Compound Injection
of Red Sage Root
(Fu fang dan shen zhu she ye)

INGREDIENTS

Red sage root (Radix Salviae Miltiorrhizae)

Dalbergia wood (Lignum Dalbergiae Odoriferae)

Injections, 2 or 5ml per ampule, 1ml contains 1g of red sage root and 1g of dalbergia wood.

EFFICACY Promoting blood circulation, removing blood stasis and improving microcirculation.

INDICATIONS Coronary heart disease and angina pectoris.

DIRECTION Intramuscular injection, 2 — 4 ml each time, 1 — 4 times a day. Intravenous injection, 4 ml each time, once a day, it can only be used after being diluted with 20ml of 50% glucose injection. Intravenous drip, 10 — 16 ml once a day, it can only be used after being diluted with 100 — 150 ml of 50% glucose injection.

Compound Semifluid Extract
of Red Sage Root
（Fu fang dan shen gao）

INGREDIENTS

Red sage root (Radix Salviae Miltiorrhizae)

Moutan bark (Cortex Moutan Radicis)

Semifluid extract, 250g or 500g per bottle.

EFFICACY Promoting blood circulation to remove blood stasis, reducing hypertension and tranquilizing the mind.

INDICATIONS Coronary heart disease, hypertension.

DIRECTION To be taken orally, 20g each time, twice a day.

Cow-bezoar Sedative Bolus
（Niu huang qing xin wan）

INGREDIENTS

Chinese yam (Rhizoma Dioscoreae)

Ginseng (Radix Ginseng)

Bighead atractylodes rhizome (Rhizoma Atractylodis Macrocephalae)

      Chinese angelica root (Radix Angelicae Sinensis)

      White peony root (Radix Paeoniae Alba)

      Artificial cow-bezoar (Calculus Bovis Facticius)

      Antelope's horn (Cornu Saigae Tataricae)

      Rhinoceros horn (Cornu Rhinocerotis)

      Musk (Moschus)

      Honeyed boluses, 3g each one, 10 boluses per box.

      EFFICACY Supplementing qi, nourishing blood, tranquilizing the mind, allaying excitement, and eliminating phlegm for resuscitation.

      INDICATIONS Stagnated heat in the chest, palpitation due to fright, fidgeting due to deficiency, vertigo, aphasia from apoplexy, deviation of the eye and mouth, hemiplegia, dysphasia and vague mind caused by deficiency of qi and blood as well as upward disturbance of phlegm and heat.

      DIRECTION To be taken orally, 1 bolus each time, or 2 boluses for serious cases, twice a day. The dose should be reduced for children.

      Contraindicated for pregnant women.

Decoction Containing Ten Ingredients
for Clearing Away Gallbladder-heat
(Shi wei wen dan tang)

INGREDIENT This prescription is formed by adding Radix Codonopsis Pilosulae, Radix Rehmanniae Praeparata, Fructus Schisandrae, Radix Polygalae and Semen Ziziphi Spinosae to and omitting Bambusae in Taeniam from the Decoction for Clearing Away Gall-bladder-Heat.

EFFICACY AND INDICATION Dispersing phlegm, tranquilizing, benefiting vital energy and nourishing blood. it is indicated for cases with palpitation, insomnia, listlessness, timidness, anorexia, fatigue, pale tongue with whitish and greasy fur, slow pulse. Both this prescription are indicated for some cases with palpitation and insomnia, but this prescription is superior for invigoration vital energy and blood and tranquilizing.

Decoction for Calming Liver-wind
(Zhen gan xi feng tang)

INGREDIENTS

Radix Achyranthis Bidentatae 30g

Haematitum 30g

Os Draconis 15g

Concha os-treae 15g

Plastrum Testudinis 15g

Radix Paeoniae Alba 15g

Radix Scrophulariae 15g

Radix Asparagi 15g

Fructus Meliae Toosendan (Pounded) 6g

Fructus Hordei Germinatus 6g

Herba Artemisiae Scopariae 6g

Radix Glycyrrhizae 3g

EFFICACY AND INDICATION Calming liver
and expelling wind; mainly for cases attributive to upward attack of liver-yang and internal stirring of liver-
wind, which are manifested as dizziness, tinnitus, or
hot sensation and pain over the head, irritability,
flushed cheeks, frequent eructation limited mobility of
limbs, deviation of the eye and mouth, or even faint-

ing, coma and paralysis, wiry and long, strong pulse.

INTERPRETATION Achyranthis Bidentatae has the effects of letting the blood flowing downward, inhibiting the hyperactive yang and nourishing liver and kidney. Haematitum has the effects of lowering the adverse rising energy, calming the liver and suppressing yang. They two used together can relieve the critical condition fo dysfunction of vital energy and blood, and are applied in large dose as the chief drugs in this prescription. Os Draconis and Concha Ostreae help Ochar to suppress yang and lower the adverse rising energy. Plastrum Testudinis, Scrophulariae, Asparagi and Paeoniae Alba are applied for nourishing liver and kidney and calming the endogenous liver-wind. Artemisiae Scopariae, Meliae Toosendan and Hordie Germinatus serve to purge liver-yang and regulate liver-energy. Glycyrrhizae acts with Hordei Germinatus to regulate the function of stomach and middle jiao, and decrease the side effects of the mineral drugs.

CLINICAL APPLICATION 1. This prescription is a common recipe for treating apoplexy resulting from exogenous wind. For cases with large amount of phlegm, omit Scrophulariae and Glycyrrhizae, add Rhizoma Arisaema cum Bile to expel wind-phlegm; for

252

cases with weak chi pulse, omit Toosendan and add Fructus Corni to nourish the liver and kidney.

2. Also applicable to cases of hypertension, cerebral thrombosis, pheochromocytoma, glaucoma, premenstrual syndrome, etc. Which are attributive to upward attack of liver-yang and internal stirring of liverwind.

Decoction for Clearing Away Gallbladder-heat
(Wen dan tang)

INGREDIENTS
Rhizoma Pinelliae 6g
Caulis Bambusae in Taeniam 6g
Fructus Autantii Immaturus(Powder-fried) 6g
Pericarpium citri Reticulatea 9g
Radix Glycyrrhizae Praeparata 5g
Poria 5g
Rhizoma Zingiberis Recens 5 pcs
Fructus Ziziphi Jujubae 1 pc
EFFICACY AND INDICATIONS Regulating the flow of qi and resolving phlegm, claering away heat

from gallbladder and regulating the stomach.

Incoordination between the gallbladder and the stomach with stirring up of phlegm-heat marked by vertigo, vomiting, gastric discomfort with acid regurgitation, palpitation, insomnia due to vexation, epilepsy, bitter taste in the mouth, slight thirst, yellow greasy fur of the tongue, and slippery, rapid pulse or taut rapid pulse.

Disorder of vegetative nerve, menopausal syndrome, neurosism, cerebral arteriosclerosis and chronic gastritis marked by the symptoms of incoordination between the gallbladder and the stomach with stirring up of phlegm-heat can be treated by the modified recipe.

Modern researches have proved that the recipe has the effects of tranquilizing the mind, coordinating the functions of vegetative nerve and arresting vomiting.

CAUTIONS Since it is a heat-clearing and phlegm-eliminating one, the recipe is not indicated for insomnia due to deficiency of heart, palpitation due to deficiency of blood, vertigo due to deficiency of yin, vomiting due to cold of the stomach, etc.

INTERPRETATION Bambusae in Taeniam can clear away gallbladder-heat, disperse phlegm and relieve vomiting; Pinelliae can dry the dampness, elimi-

254

nate sputum, regulate the stomach and relieve vomiting. They both serve as the chief drugs of the prescription. Aurantii Immaturus is applied for promoting the circulation of vital energy and discharging sputum; Citri Grandis for regulating vital energy and drying dampness; Poria for strengthening the spleen and promoting diuresis. Zingiberis Recens is helpful for dispersing sputum and inhibits the toxicity of Pinelliae. A small amount of Glycyrrhizae and Ziziphi Jujubae are used to benefit the spleen and regulate the stomach.

Decoction for Elimination Dampness and Relieving Rheumatism (Chu shi juan bi tang)

INGREDIENTS

Rhizoma Atractylodis 12g

Rhizoma Atractylodis Macrocephalae 10g

Poria 10g

Rhizoma seu Radix Notopterygii 10g

Rhizoma Alismatis 10g

Exocarpium Citri Grandis 6g

Radix Glycyrrhizae 3g

Succus Zingiberis 3 spoonfuls

Succus Bambusae 3 spoonfuls

EFFICACY AND INDICATION Strengthening the spleen, eliminating dampness, expelling wind, dissipating phlegm, relieving rheumatism and alleviating pain; mainly for cases of rheumatism manifested as localized arthralgia which will be aggravated in rainy days, fatigue, white and greasy fur on the tongue, wiry and smooth pulse, which are attributive to retention of dampness in the speen and stomach and attack of wind-phlegm to the meridians and joints.

INTERPRETATION Atractylodis acts as the chief drug in the prescription and is applied in large dosage, which has the effects of activating the spleen, drying demapness, eliminating wind and alleviating pain. Atractylodis Macrocephalae and Poria serve to strengthen the spleen and promote diuresis. Citri Grandis can regulate vital energy and activate the spleen, thus assists in eliminating dampness. Succus Zingiberis and Lophatheri are used to expel wind, dredge meridians and dissipate phlegm, and the cold and spleen-damaging effect of Lophatheri is avoided by the simultaneous application of Succus Zingiberis and Atractylodis. Glycyrrhizae serves to regulate the other drugs.

CLINICAL APPLICATION 1. For cases of apoplexy manifested as distortion of the face, dysphasia, numbness and spasms of limbs, or even hemiplegia, white and greasy fur on the tongue, wiry and smooth pulse, which are attributive to the attack of meridians by phlegm-dampness, omit Glycyrrhizae and add Scorpio, Bombyx Batryticatus.

2. For cases attributive to the attack of upper orifices by phlegm-dampness, which manifest as vertigo accompanied with nausea, vomiting, tinnitus, deafness, white and greasy tongue fur and wiry pulse, add Rhizoma Pinelliae Praeparate, rhizoma Gastrodiae and omit Glycyrrhizae.

3. Also applicable to cases with rheumatic arthritis, sciatica and beriberi attributive to accmulation of dampness in the spleen and stomach; to cases of facial paralysis, poliomyelitis and thromboangiitis obliterans of cerebral vessels with hemiplesia attributive to attack of meridians by wind-phlegm; and to cases of hypertension and cerebral arteriosclerosis, with dizziness attributive to attack of the upper orifices by phlegm-dampness.

Decoction for Fluid
Increasing and Purgation
(Zeng ye cheng qi tang)

INGREDIENTS
Radix Rehmanniae 25g
Radix Scrophulariae 25g
Radix Ophiopogonis 15g
Radix et Rhizoma Rhei 9g
Natrii Sulfas 5g

EFFICACY AND INDICATIONS Nourishing yin to promote the production of body fluid, inducing the bowel movement to expel the heat evil; mainly for constipation attributive to the accumulation of heat evil and consumption of yin-fluid.

Applicable to cases of gingivitis with red and uncoated tongue, which are attributive to yin-deficiency and fire hyperactivity. Also applicable to cases of intestinal tuberculosis, chronic pancreatitis, hemorrhoids, etc. with constipation attributive to yin-deficiency and accumulation of heat evil; to cases of periodontitis, hypertension, glaucoma, etc. with toothache or headache attributive to yin-deficiency and fire hyperactivity.

INTERPRETATION Rhei and Natrii sulfas are purgatives, but they may aggravate the deficiency of body fluid and fail to induce bowel movement in case of constipation due to lack of body fluid. So Rehmanniae, Scrophulariae and Ophiopogonis are used in large dose for promoting the production of body fluid and nourishing yin, and the purgative effects of Rhei and Natrii sulfas are ensured.

Decoction for Lengthening Age and Relieving Aphasia (Zi shou jie yu tang)

INGREDIENT
Radix Ledeboruiellae 10g
Radix Aconiti Praeparata 10g
Rhizoma Gastrodiae 10g
Semen Zizphi spinosae 10g
Cornu Saigae Tataricae 3g
Ramulus Cinnamomi 8g
Rhizoma seu Radix Notopterygii 8g
Radix Glycyrrhizae 8g

Succus Rotundus (Mixed with the decoction) 20g

Succus Zingiberis Recens (Mixed with the decoction) 10g

EFFICACY Warming the spleen, dispersing phlegm, suppressing wind and waking the patients from unconsciousness; mainly for cases of apoplexy attributive to dysfunction of spleen-yang, accumulation of phlegm-dampness in the interior, attack of wind and obstruction of the upper orifices, which manifest as hemiplegia, stiff tongue, aphasia, white and greasy fur on the tongue, floating and smooth pulse.

INTERPRETATION Ledebouriellae and Notopterygii expel the wind from outside, while gastrodiae and Cornu saigae Tataricae suppress the wind inside the body. the four drugs act together to get rid of all exogenous and endogenous wind. Aconiti Praeparata, Ramulus Cinnamomi and Glycyrrhizae serve to warm spleen-yang and disperse phlegm-dampness. Succus Bambusae and succus Zingiberis Recens are applied for expelling wind-phlegm and opening the orifices. Ziziphi Jujubae is a tranquilizing agent, when used together with Succus Zingiberis Recens it restores the ability of speaking.

CLINICAL APPLICATION 1. For cases of stiff

260

tongue with aphasia attributive to declination of kidney-yang and obstruction of the orifices by adverse rising phlegm-dampness, this prescription is not suitable and Decoction of Rehmanniae should be applied.

2. Applicable to the initial stage of tetanus attributive to stagnation of wind-phlegm in the meridians, which manifest as aversion to cold, fever, trismus, stiffness of neck and back, spasm of limbs, profuse expectoration, white and greasy fur on the tongue, wiry and tense pulse.

3. Also applicable to cases of cerebral thrombosis, thromboangiitis obliterans, hypertensive cerebral disease and rheumatic cerebroangiitis marked by hemiplegia and aphasis, which are attributive to the obsturction of the upper orifices by phlegm-dampness.

Decoction for Nourishing
the Liver and Kidney
(Yi guan jian)

INGREDIENTS
Radix Glehniae 10g
Radix Ophiopogonis 10g

Radix Angelicae Sinensis 10g

Radix rehmanniae 30g

Fructus Lycii 10g

Fructus Mediae Toosendan 5g

EFFICACY AND INDICATIONS Nourishing the liver and kidney, soothing the liver and regulating the circulation of qi.

Hypochondriac and thoracic pain due to deficiency of yin of the liver and kidney with stagnancy of the liver-qi, manifested by hypochondriac and thoracic fullness and pain, acid regurgitation, dry mouth and throat, reddened tongue with reduced saliva, thready and feeble or feeble and taut pulse, as well as hernia and abdominal mass.

Moreover, other cases attributed to deficiency of yin of the liver and kidney such as chronic hepatitis, primary stage of cirrhosis, fatty liver, chronic gastritis, gastric ulcer, diabetes, hypertension as well as other chronic disorders can respond well to the treatment with the modified recipe.

Modern studies have confirmed that this recipe has the efficacies of protecting the liver, lowering the level of blood sugar, strengthening immunity, tranquilizing the mind, relieving inflammation, allaying fever, arresting pain, regulating vegetative nerve, etc.

CAUTIONS Since there are more greasy drugs for nourishment in the recipe, it is better not to be administered for those with sputum and stagnation of body fluid.

INTERPRETATION Being the largest in dosage, Radix Rehmanniae is preferred to as a principal drug used to tonify the insufficiency of genuine yin of the liver and kindey by way of nourishing yin and enriching the blood. Glehnia root, Ophiopogon root, Chinese angelica root and Wolfberry fruit, possessing the effects of supplementing yin and soothing the liver, share the part of an assistant drug along with Radix Rehmanniae which has the effects of nourishing yin, enriching the blood and promoting the production of body fluid. Functioning as an adjuvant and guiding drug, Sichuan Chinaberry is used in small amount to sooth the liver and regulate the circulation of qi, and though bitter and dry in property, its dry property can be restrained and the effect of relieving the depressed liver remained when it is decocted together with a large amount of yin-tonifying drugs with a sweet flavor and cold property.

Decoction for Removing Blood Stasis in the Chest
(Xue fu zhu yu tang)

INGREDIENTS

Semen Presicae 10g

Radix Angelicae Sinensis 10g

Radix Paeoniae Rubra 10g

Radix Achyranthis Bidentatae 10g

Flos Carthami 6g

Rhizoma Ligustici Chuanxiong 6g

Radix Bupleuri 6g

Fructus Aurnatii 6g

Radix Rehmanniae 15g

Radix Platycodi 3g

Radix Glycyrrhizae 3g

All the drugs listed above are to be decocted in water for oral administration.

EFFICACY AND INDICATION Activating blood circulation to remove blood atasis, promoting the circulation of vital energy and relieving pain; mainly for cases of retention of blood stasis in the chest, manifested as localized and stabbing pain over the chest, dark,reddish tongue, wiry and tense or unsmooth pulse.

INTERPRETATION Angelicae Sinensis, Persicae, Ligustici Chuanxiong, Carthami, Achyranthis Bidentatae have the effects of activating blood circulation and removing blood stasis, and are usually applied for stagnation of blood flow. Bupleuri, Aurantii, Platycodi ease the chest and promote the circulation of vital energy and blood. Rehmanniae and Angelicae Sinensis have the effects of nourishing blood and activating blood circulation so as to avoid consumption of yin-blood when blood-stasis removing drugs are used. They help Persicae and Achyranthis Bidentatae to promote bowel novement and let the blood flowing downward. glycyrrhizae regulates the above drugs.

CLINICAL APPLICATION 1. For cases of amenorrhea and dysmenorrhea due to blood stasis, omit Glycyrrhizae and Platycodi from this prescription, and add Rhizoma Cyperi and Herba Leonuri to regulate menstruation, and relieve pain.

2. Also applicable to cases of chest contusion, cerebral thrombosis, hypertension, cirrhosis of liver, thromboangiitis obliterans, rheumatic heart disease and coronary heart disease with chest pain which are attributive to retention of blood stasis in the chest or ob-

265

struction of blood stasis with stagnation of vital energy.

Decoction of Antelope's Horn and Uncaria Stem
(Ling jiao gou teng tang)

INGREDIENTS

cornu Saigae Tataricae (decocted first)4. 5g

Ramulus Uncariae cum Uncis (decocted later)9g

Folium Mori 6g

Bulbus Fritillariae Cirrhosae 12g

Radix Rehmanniae 15g

Caulis Bambusae in Taenis (Fresh and prepared,
decocted first in water)9g

Flos Chrysanthemi 9g

Radix Paeoniae Alba 9g

Poria cum Ligno Hospite 9g

Radix Glycyrrhizae Recens 3g

EFFICACY AND INDICATIONS Removing
pathogenic heat from the liver and calming endogenous
wind and increasing body fluid to relax muscles and
tendons. Occurrence of wind syndrome in case of extreme heat marked by persistent high fever, listlessness

and convulsion, or coma in serious case, dry and deep-red tongue, or prickled and parched tongue, taut and rapid pulse.

Hypertension, functional disturbance of vegetative nerve cerebrovascular accident, hyperthyroidism, epilepsy and vertigo marked by occurrence of wind syndrome in case of extreme heat can be treated by the modified recipe.

INTERPRETATION Cornu Saigae Tataricae and Ramulus Uncariae cum Uncis have the effects of clearing away heat evil, cooling the liver, calming wind and relieving spasm, and serve as the chief drugs in this prescription. Mori and Chrysanthemi are helpful to expel wind-heat from the liver channel. Since severe heat is liable to consume yin-fluid, Paeoniae Alba, glycyrrhizae and rehmanniae are applied to nourish yin increase the production of body fluid. Fritillariae Cirrhosae and Caulis bambusae in Taeniam serve to clear away heat and disperse phlegm. Poria is applied for tranquilizing.

Decoction of Bupleuri for
Regulating Shaoyang and Yangming
(Da chai hu tang)

INGREDIENTS

Radix Bupleuri 9g

Radix Scutellariae 9g

Radix Paeoniae Alba 9g

Rhizoma Pinelliae praeparata 9g

Fructus Aurantii Immaturus 9g

Radix et Rhizoma Rhei 6g

Fructus Ziziphi Jujubae 4Pcs

Phizoma Zingiberis Recens 12g

EFFICACY Regulating shaoyang and purging the stagnation of heat evil; mainly for shaoyang and yangming syndrome complex, manifested as alternating episodes of chills and fever, epigastric pain, vomiting, constipation or diarrhea, yellow fur on the tongue, wiry and strong pulse.

INDICATION 1. For cases accompanied with jaundice, omit Zingiberis Recens, Ziziphi Jujubae and add Herba Artemisiae Scopariae, Cortex Phellodendri to clear away heat evil, eliminate dampness evil, and relieve jaundice.

2. For cases attributive to upward attack of liver-fire and gallbladder-fire, manifested as headache,, tinnitus, conjunctivitis, red tongue with yellow fur, wiry and rapid pulse.

3. Also applicable to cases of acute cholecystitis, acute pancreatitis, intestinal obstruction, etc., which are attributive to shaoyang and yangming syndrome complex, or sthenia-heat of gallbladder and stomach; also to cases of hypertension, acute conjunctivitis, etc. attributive to upward attack of liver-fire and gallbladder-fire.

INTERPRETATION This prescription is composed of the principal drugs of Decoction of Bupleuri for Regulating Shaoyang and Decoction for Mild Purgation. Radix Ginseng used in the former is for tonifying middle jiao and supporting the healthy energy to prevent the pathogenic factor invading further to the interior. As the pathogenic factor has invaded yangming and the sthenic heat-syndrome of yang.ning such as constipation, abdominal pain and yellow fur has appeared, tonics may hinder the elimination of pathogenic factor, so Ginseng and Radix Glycyrrhizae are omitted. Decoction for Mild Purgation is designed for the

269

treatment of yangming hollow-organ sthenia-syndrome, Cortex Magnoliae Officinalis is omitted in case of absence of significant abdominal fullness. Paeoniae Alba is added to disperse the depressed liver-energy and alleviate pain when it acts with Bupleuri and Aurantii Immaturus and may be beneficial to abdominal pain caused by gall-energy attacking the stomach.

Decoction of Coptidis and Colla Corii Asini
(Huang lian e jiao tang)

INGREDIENTS
Rhizoma Coptidis 10g
Radix Scutellariae 10g
Colla Corii Asini (dissolved) 12g
Radix Paeoniae Alba 12g
A fresh Egg Yolk (mixed)
EFFICACY AND INDICATIONS clearing away heart-fire and nourishing kidney yin; mainly for cases attributive to damage of ture-yin by the heat evil entering shaoyin and hyperactivity of heart-fire, which are manifested as vexation, sleeplessness, feverish sensa-

tion over the body, palms and soles, dry mouth and throat, oliguria with yellow urine, red or crimson tongue with yellow fur, small and rapid pulse. For cases with fresh blood in the stool, irritability, dry throat, bitter mouth, red tongue with yellow fur, small and rapid pulse, which are attributive to excess of yang-energy and deficiency of yin-energy, and damage of the vessels by heat, use Radix Rehmanniae instead of egg yolk to cool the blood, stop bleeding and nourish yin-fluid.

Also applicable to cases of hyperthyroidism, diabetes mellitus, hypertension, neurasthenia, etc. with insomnia or nocturnal emission, and cases of nonspecific proctitis, tuberculous ulceration of rectum, chronic bacillary dysentery, etc., with bloody stool, which are attributive to excess of yang-energy and deficiency of yin-energy.

For cases with nocturnal emission or praecox ejaculation accompanied with dizziness, irritability, insomnia, oliguria with yellw urine, red tongue, small and repid pulse, which are attributive to hyperactivity of fire evil and insufficiency of water, apply Cortex Phellodendri instead of Scutellariae to clear away the prime-minister fire and nourish kidney-yin.

Decoction of Gastrodia
and Uncaria
(Tian ma gou teng yin)

INGREDIENTS
Rhizoma Gastrodiae 9g
Ramulus Uncariae Cum Uncis (decocted later)
12g
Concha Haliotidis (decocted first) 18g
Fructus Gardeniae 9g
Radix Scutellariae 9g
Radix Achyranthis Bidentatae 12g
Cortex Eucommiae 9g
Herba Leonuri 9g
Ramulus Loranthi 9g
Caulis Polygoni Multiflori 9g
Poria cum Lingo Hospite 9g

EFFICACY AND INCICATIONS Calming the liver to stop endogenous wind, clearing away pathogenic heat, promoting blood circulation and nourishing the liver and kidney. Wind-syndromes caused by hyperactivity of the liver-yang marked by headache, vertigo, tinnitus and dim eyesight, involuntary movement of limbs, insomnia, or even hemiplegia, red tongue, taut and rapid pulse.

Hypertension, functional disturbance of vegetative nerve, cerebrovascular accident, hyperthyroidism, epilepsy and vertigo marked by wind-syndrome caused by hyperactivity of the liver-yang can be treated by the modified recipe.

INTERPRETATION Rhizoma Gastrodiae, Ramulus Vncariae Cum Vncis and Concha Haliotidis calm the liver to stop the wind as principal drugs. Fructus Gardeniae and Radix Scutellariae clear away heat and purge fire from the liver channel as assistant drugs. Herba Leonuri promotes blood circulation and induces diuresis. Radix Achyranthis Bidentatae ensures proper downward flow of the blood from the head. Cortex Eucommiae and Ramulus Loranthi nourish the liver and kidney. Csulis Polygoni Multiflori and Poria cum Ligno Hospite tranquilize the mind. The drugs mentioned above are used as adjuvant and guiding drugs.

Modern researches have proved that the recipe has the effects of tranquilizing the mind, relieving spasm, resisting epilepsy, dilating blood vessels and lowering high blood pressure. It also has the fever-allaying, antibacterial and antiinflammatory effects.

Decoction of Gentianae for
Purging Liver-fire
（Long dan xie gan tang）

INGREDIENTS
Herba Gentianae (fried with vine) 6g
Radix Bupleuri 6g
Radix Glycyrrhizae 6g
Rhizoma Alismatis 10g
Semen Plantaginis 10g
Caulis Akebiae 10g
Radix Rehmanniae (crude) 10g
Fructus Gardeniae (fried) 10g
Radix Scutellariae (fried)10g
Radix Angelicae Sinensis(mixed with wine) 3g

EFFICACY AND INDICATION Purging the
sthenia fire of liver and gallbladder, clearing away the
dampness-heat evil from triple jiao; mainly for cases
with flaming up of sthenia fire in the liver and gallbladder, manifested as headache, hypochondriac pain, bitter taste in the mouth, congestion of the conjunctiva

274

and deafness, and for cases with downward attack of dampness-heat from the liver and gallbladder, manifested as stranguria with turbid urine, pruritus vulvae and leukorrhagia.

INTERPRETATION Gentianae, Scutellariae and Gardeniae have the effects of purging sthenia fire in the liver and gallbladder and clearing away dampness -heat from the lower jiao. Caulis Akebiae, Alismatis and Plantaginis have the effects of clearing away the dampness-heat evil from the lower jiao and leading the fire out through urination. Angelicae Sinensis together with Rehmanniae are used for nourishing yin and blood, and preventing the heat evil damage the liver-yin. Bupleuri is used for activating the liver and gallbladder without damaging the liver-yin when it is applied with Glycyrrhizae. The combination of above drugs constitutes, a prescription exerting both prging and tonic, nourishing and clearing effects, so that the liver-fire can be purged and dampness-heat can be cleared away.

INDICATION 1. For cases of jaundice attributive to dampness-heat attacking the liver and gallbladder, omit Glycyrrhizae and Rehmanniae and add Herba Artemisiae Scopariae and Radix et Rhizoma Rahei to eliminate the heat evil through urination and defecation.

2. For cases of leukorrhagia, with yellow or red and white, thick, foul discharge, red tongue with yellowish and greasy fur, smooth and rapid pulse, which are attributive to downward attack of dampness-heat from the liver channel, omit Glycyrrhizae and use Cortex Phellodendri instead of Scutellariae.

3. Also applicable to cases of acute conjunctivitis, acute otitis media, furuncle of the vestibulum nasi and external auditory canal, hypertension which are attributive to flaming up of sthenia fire in the liver and gallbladder; to cases of icteric hepatitis, cholecystitis, herpes zoster which are attributive to retention of dampness-heat evil in the liver and gallbladdrt; to cases of urinary infection, pelvic inflammation, prostatitis, which are attributive to downward attack of dampness-heat evil from the liver and gallbladder.

Decoction of Persicae
for Purgation
(Tao he cheng qi tang)

INGREDIENTS

Semen Persicae 12g

Radix et Rhizoma Rhei 12g

Ramulus Cinnamomi 10g

Radix Glycyrrhizae Praeparata 6g

Natrii Sulfas (taken after mixing with decoction)
6g

EFFICACY Eliminating blood stasis and purging
heat evil; for blood stagnation syndrome due to accumulation of blood stasis and heat evil in the lower jiao,
which is manifested as distending pain over the lower
abdomen, irritability, sunken and solid pulse.

INTERPRETATION Persicae has the effects of
activating blood circulation to eliminate blood stasis,
and also lubricating the intestine to promote bowel
movement. Rhei, here to be decocted simultaneously,
is used not only for moving bowel movement and purging heat, but also for activating blood circulation and e-
liminating blood stasis. Thus, two drugs used together
have the effects of eliminating blood stasis and clearing
away heat evil. Ramulus cinnamomi of acrid-warm nature, when used together with large dosage of Rhei,
acts downward to activate blood circulation and dredge
the vessels instead of eliminating superficial evils as
usual. Natrii Sulfas helps Rhei to promote bowel move-

ment and clear away heat evil, their potent purgative actions are inhibited by Ramulus Cinnamomi and Glycyrrhizae.

INDICATION 1. For cases of preceded menstrual cycle, amenorrhea, metrorrhagia, etc. , attributive to combination of blood stasis and heat evil in the lower jiao, omit Glycyrrhizae from this prescription and add Radix Angelicae sinensis to regulate menstruation, activate blood circulation, eliminate blood stasis and stop bleeding.

2. For cases of abdominal pain after operat on due to blood stasis, or trauma (especially the early stage of fractures of thoracic or lumbar vertebrae), which are attributive to combination of blood stasis and heat evil, omit Glycyrrhizae and add Radix Cyathulae to activate blood circulation and eliminate blood stasis, and let the blood flowing downwards.

3. Applicable to cases of hematemesis, headache, congestion of conjunctiva, which are attributive to upward attack of blood stasis and heat evil.

4. Also applicable to cases of intestinal obstruction, pelvic cellulitis, appendicitis, etc. with abodominal pain, or cases of retention of placenta, functional uterine bleeding. etc. with vaginal bleeding, or cases of

hypertension, periodontitis, etc. with headache or bleeding from the gum, which are attributive to combination or upward attack of blood stasis and heat evil.

Decoction of Pinelliae, Atractylodis Macrocephalae and Gastrodiae
(Ban xia bai zhu tain ma tang)

INGREDIENTS
Rhizoma Pinelliae 10g
Rhizoma Gastrodiae 10g
Poria 10g
Rhizoma Atractylodis Macrocephalae 12g
Exocarpium Citri Grandis 6g
Radix Glycyrrhizae 2g
Rhizoma Zingiberis Recens 3 pcs
Fructus Ziziphi Jujubae 2 pcs
EFFICACY Dispersing phlegm, calming wind, strengthening the spleen and eliminating dampness; mainly for wind-phlegm syndrome attributive to production of phlegm by dampness in the speen and the attack of endogenous liver-wind, which is manifested as

dizziness, headache, heaviness of the head, feeling of oppression over the chest, nausea, vomiting, profuse expectoration of thick sputum, white and greasy fur on the tongue, wiry and smooth pulse, etc.

INTERPRETATION The combination of Pinelliae and Gastrodiae is an effective Remedy for dizziness and headache attributive to wind-phlegm. Atractylodis Macrocephalae and Poria are applied to strengthen spleen and expel dampness. Citri Grandis serves to regulate vital energy and disperse phlegm, and also enhance the effects of Pinelliae. When used together with Atractylodis Macrocephalae and Poria, it can strengthen and promote the function of spleen and stomach, so as to inhibit the production of phlegm. Zingiberis Recens accompanied with Gastrodiae can enhance the effects of dispersing phlegm and calming wind, and also decrease the toxicity of the latter. Glycyrrhizae and Ziziphi Jujubae act with Atractylodis Macrocephalae and Poria to strengthen the spleen and stomach. This prescription is designed for calming endogenous wind especially by eliminating phlegm.

INDICATION 1. For cases of stroke manifested as sudden onset of coma, lockjaw, salivation, white and greasy fur on the tongue, wiry and smooth pulse, which are attributive to obstruction of orifices by wind-phlegm, Bolus of Resina Liquidambaris Orienstalis should be applied first and then followed by this prescription. In this case omit Glycyrrhizae and Ziziphi Jujubae, and add Rhizoma Arisaema cum Bile and Rhizoma Acori Graminei.

2. Also applicable to cases of Meniere's syndrome, cerebral artherosclerosis, epilepsy, etc., marked by dizziness attributive to wind-phlegm.

Decoction of Rhei
and Moutan Radicis
(Da huang mu dan tang)

INGREDIENTS
Radix et Rhizoma Rhei 12g
Cortex Moutan Radicis 12g
Semen Persicae 10g
Semen Benincasae 30g
Natrii Sulfas 9g
EFFICACY Clearing away heat evil and relaxing bowel movement; promoting blood circulation and promoting subsidence of swelling; mainly for the early

stage of acute appendicitis manifested as pain and tenderness over the right lower abdomen, limited extension of the right hip, fever, smooth and rapid pulse.

INDICATION 1. For cases affected by potent heat-toxic evil with yellowish and dryness fur on the tongue, add Herba Violae or Herba Hydyotis Diffusae to clear away heat evil and detoxicate.

2. For cases of periappendicular abscess, add Spina Gleditsiae and Radix Angelicae Sinensis to activate the blood circulation, promote the subsidence of swelling, perforation and pus drainage.

3. Also applicable to cases of adnexitis with abdominal pain and fever attributed to accumulation of blood stasis and heat.

4. Also applicable to cases of hypertension, which is attributive to sthenia-syndrome.

INTERPRETATION Rhei has not only the effects of clearing away the heat evil and moving the bowels, but als of promoting blood circulation and removing blood stasis (that is why it needs not to be decocted later). Moutan Radicis has the similar effect as that of Rhei, but it can cool the blood instead of moving the bowels. They act as principal drugs in this prescription to dredge the heat stagnated in the intestine.

Natrii Sulfas has the effects of softening the hard lumps and dispersing the stagnation, and enhance the purgative effect of Rhei. Persicae is good for removing blood stasis, and helps Moutan Radicis to promote blood circulation. Benincasae has the effect of dispersing the stagnation and promoting the subsidence of carbuncle when the pus is not formed and also promoting pus drainage when the pus is formed.

Docoction of
Uncariae cum Uncis
(Gou teng yin)

INGREDIENTS

Ramulus Uncariae cum Uncis 12g

Cornu Saigae Tataricae (decocted first)6g

Rhizoma Gastrodiae 6g

Radix Pseudostellariae 6g

Scorpio (detoxified) 3 pcs

Radix Glycyrrhizae 3g

EFFICACY AND INDICATIONS Clearing away heat, suppressing wind, supporting healthy energy and expelling evil; mainly for acute cases of infants manifested as high fever, palpitation, convulsion, lockjaw, fixation of eyes, red or crimson tongue, rapid pulse, which are attributive to hyperactivity of heat with production of wind.

Applicable to eclampsia of pregnancy with red and uncoated tongue, wiry and rapid pulse, which is attributive to upward attack of liver-yang. Also indicated for cases with dizziness, flushed cheeks, which are attributive to attack of the orifices by the hyperactive liver-fire. Also applicable to cases of common cold, malaria, etc. with high fever and convulsion attributive to hyperactivity of heat with production of wind; and to cases of hypertension, Meniere's syndrome, etc. with dizziness attributive to hyperactivity of liver-fire.

INTERPREIATION Uncariae cum Uncis can clear away heat, to expel wind and relieve spasm, but its action is relatively mild. For cases with high fever and convulsion, Cornu Saigae Tataricae should be applied as well. Gastrodiae used together with Scorpio can also expel wind and relieve spasm. Since the course of disease in infants is liable to be changed, Pseudostellariae and Glycyrrhizae are applied to prevent the damage of vital energy and consumption of body fluid.

Gastrodia Tuber Bolus
(Tian ma wan)

INGREDIENTS

Gastrodia tuber (Rhizoma Gastrodiae)

Notopterygium (Rhizoma seu Radix Notopterygii)

Pubescent angelica root (Radix Angelicae Pubescentis)

Eucommia bark (Cortex Eucommiae)

Achyranthes root (Radix Achyranthis Bidentatae)

Hypoglauca yam (Rhizoma Dioscoreae Hypoglaucae)

Prepared aconite root (Radix Aconiti Lateralis Praeparata)

Chinese angelica root (Radix Angelicae Sinensis)

Rehmannia root (Radix Rehmanniae)

Scrophularia root (Radix Scrophulariae)

Grind the above drugs into fine powder, mix it with honey and make them into boluses, 9g each bolus, 10 boluses per box.

EFFICACY Expelling wind and removing dampness, relaxing muscles and tendons and activating the flow of qi and blood in the channels and collaterals, promoting blood circulation to relieve pain.

INDICATIONS Symptoms due to apoplexy involving the channels such as stiff limbs, numb hands and feet, lassitude and pain in the loins and legs, difficulty in walking. And rheumatic arthritis and hemiplegia caused by sequel of stroke.

DIRECTION To be taken orally, 1 bolus each time, once or twice a day.

It should be carefully administered to pregnant women.

Jianling Decoction
（Jian ling tang）

INGREDIENTS
Rhizoma Dioscoreae
Radix Achyranthis Bidentatae
Ochra
Os Draconis
Concha Ostreae
Radix Rehmanniae
Radix Paeoniae Alba and Semen Biotae

EFFICACY Suppressing the liver-yang and calming wind.

INDICATION It is indicated for cases attributive to upper attack of liver-yang, which are manifested as dizziness, tinnitus, irritability, insomnia, wiry and long pulse. This prescription has a stronger effect for calming the sthenic yang; while Decoction of Cornu Saigae Tatarica and Uncariae cum Uncis has a stronger effect for clearing away heat, and is more suitable for cases of high fever and convulsion due to hyperactivity of heat and stirring of wind.

Jiaotai Bolus
(Jiao tai wan)

INGREDIENTS
Rhizoma Coptidis
Cortex Cinnamomi
EFFICACY Clearing away the heat-evil located at heart, and keeping heart-fire and kidney-water in balance; mainly for cases attributive to insufficiency of heart-energy and imbalance between heart-fire and kid-

ney-water, which are manifested as dreamfulness, timidness, palpitation, insomnia.

INDICATION The action of this prescription and Pill for Calming the Mental State (An shen ding zhi wan) is similar.

1. Applicable to cases after epileptic attack manifested as spiritlessness, palpitation, shortness of breath, anorexia, profuse expectoration, pale tongue with whitish fur, small and smooth pulse, which are attributive to insufficiency of heart-energy and stagnation of phlegm in the heart orifice.

2. Also indicated for cases of nocturnal emission attributive to imbalance between heart-fire and kidney-water.

3. Also applicable to cases of sinus bradycardia, atrioculoventricular block, sinus arrhythmia, vegetative nervous dysfunction, hypertension, neurasthenia, etc. marked by palpitation, insomnia, or noctarnal emission, which are attributive to insufficiency of heart-energy and imbalance between heartr-fire and kidney-water.

4. The Pill for Calming the Mental State is more suitable for cases attributive to insufficiency of heart-energy, while Jiaotai Pill is suitable for cases attributive

to hyperactivity of heart-fire.

Pill for Calming the Mental state
(An shen ding zhi wan)

INGREDIENTS

Radix Codonopsis Pilosulae 12g

Poria 12g

Lignum Pini Poriaferum 12g

Dens Draconis 20g

Radix Polygalae 6g

Rhizoma Acori Graminei 6g

INDICATIONS Nourishing heart, calming mental state, and keeping heart-fire and kidney-water in balance; mainly for cases attributive to insufficiency of heart-energy and imbalance between heart-fire and kidney-water, which are manifested as dreamfulness, timidness, palpitation, insomnia, pale tongue, small and weak pulse.

1. Applicable to cases after epileptic attack manifested as spiritlessness, palpitation, shortness of breath, anorexia, profuse expectoration, pale tongue with whitish fur, small and smooth pulse, which are

attributive to insufficiency of heart-energy and stagnation of phlegm in the heart orifice.

2. Also indicated for cases of nocturnal emission attributive to imbalance between heart-firt and kidney-water.

3. Also applicable to cases of sinus bradycardia, atrioculoventricular block, sinus arrhythmia, vegetative nervous dysfunction, neurasthenia, etc. marked by palpitation, insomnia, or nocturnal emission, which are attributive to insufficiency of heart-energy and imbalance between heart-fire and kidney-water.

INTERPRETATION Codonopsis Pilosulae, Poria, Lignum Pini Poriaferum and Dens Draconis have the effects of invigorating heart-energy and calming mental state. Polygalae and Graminei are applied for opening the heart orifice and serve to balance heart-fire and kidney-water when used together with Dens Draconis.

Pill for Controlling Fluid
(Gong di wan)

INGREDIENTS

Radix Rehmanniae Praeparata 20g

Semen Cuscutae 15g

Rhizoma Atractylodis Macrocephalae 15g

Fructus Psoraleae 15g

Fructus Alpiniae Oxyphyllae 10g

Fructus Schisandrae 10g

Radix Aconiti Praeparata 10g

Poria 10g

Rhizoma Dioscoreae 10g

Semen Allii Tuberosi 10g

EFFICACY; Tonifying kidney, relieving nocturnal emission, strengthening spleen and controlling fluid; mainly for cases attributive to declination of kidney-yang and failure of controlling fluid by the urinary bladder, which manifest as incontinence of urine, or enuresis, or nocturia, tiredness, intolerance of cold, dizziness, lumbago, weakness of lower limbs, pale tongue with white and smooth fur, sunken and weak pulse.

INTERPRETATION Aconiti Praeparata, Allii Tuberosi, Cuscutae and Psoraleae have the effects of tonifying kidney-yand and relieving nocturnal emission. Rehmanniae Praeparata also can invigorate kidney-yang and increase essence production. Alpiniae Oxyphyllae is used for invigorating kidney and preserving essence, and Schisandrae for strengthening kidney and controlling vital energy; they two act together to control urination and stop enuresis. Atractylodis Macrocephalae, Dioscoreae and Poria serve to strengthen the spleen and, in turn, to control water discharge.

INDICATION 1. Applicable to cases of leucorrhagia with profuse, thin discharge, lumbago, cold feeling over the lower abdomen, nocturia, pale tongue with white fur, slow pulse, which are attributive to deficiency of kidney-yang, dysfunction of dai channel and downward loss of fouyid.

2. Also indicated for cases of diabetes involving the lower jiao characterized by polyuria, polydipsia, blackish complexion, dryness of external ears, emaciation, fatigue, pale tongue with white fur, sunken, small and weak pulse, which are attriburive to insufficiency of both kidney-yin and kidney-yang.

3. Also applicable to cases of chronic renal tubular dysfunction, hypertensive renal disease, primary aldosteronism, endometriosis and senile vaginitis, which are attributive to declination of kidney-ying, and to cases of diabetes insipidus, psychic polyuria and polydipsia, which are attributive to insufficiency of both kidney-yin and didney-ying.

292

Pill for Lubricating Intestine
(Run chang wan)

INGREDIENTS

Cauda Radix Angelicae Sinensis 10g

Rhizoma seu Radix Notopterygii 10g

Radix et Rhizoma Rhei 10g

Semen Persicae 10g

Fructus Cannabis 30g

Mel 30g

EFFICACY AND INDICATIONS Activating blood circulation, expelling wind, lubrication intestines and promoting bowel movement; mainly for cases of constipation accompanied with dizziness, wiry and small, rapid pulse, which are attributive to involvement of the lung and the intestine by liver-wind and consumption of body fluid.

Applicable to cases of constipation occurring in the initial stage of trauma of lumbar vertebrae, such as prolapse of lumbar intervertebral disc, compressed fracture of lumber vertebra, etc.

Also applicable to sequelae of cerebrovascular accidents and hypertension with constipation attributive to attact of the lung by liver-wind.

In the prescription, Notopterygii may be replaced by Radix Gentianae Macrophyllae and Radix Ledebouriellae which are antiwind drugs with lubricating action. They can eliminate wind but do not consume body fluid.

INTERPRETATION Cauda Radix Angelicae Sinensis combined with Notopterygii and Cannabis serves to activate blood circulation, soothe the liver, suppress wind and promote bowel movement. Persicae and Rhei, when used together with Cauda Radix Angelicae Sinensis, can activate blood circulation, remove blood stasis, lubricate the intestine, promote blwel movement, and clear away heat. Mel enhances the intestine-lubricating effect of the above drugs. Notopterygii can eliminate wind, its drying nature is counteracted by Cannabis and the laxative effect of which is enhanced by the former. In sum, the prescription has a strong effect for lubricating the intestine and promoting bowel movement, and is used as a symptomatic remedy.

Pill for Purging Liver-fire
(Xie qing wan)

INGREDIENTS

Radix Gentianae 10g

Radix et Rhizoma Rhei 9g

Fructus Gardeniae 9g

Radix Angelicae Sinensis 6g

Rhizoma Ligustici Chuanxiong 6g

Radix Ledebouriellae 6g

Rhizoma et Radix Notopterygii 6g

Herba Lophatheri 2g

EFFICACY Purging Liver-fire; mainly for cases attributive to stagnation of liver-fire, which are manifested as conjunctivitis, irritability, discharge of reddish urine, constipation, red tongue with yellow fur, bounding and solid pulse.

INDICATIONS Indicated for cases attributive to flaming up of liver-fire, which are manifested as headache at the temporal regions, dizziness, listlessness, insomnia, red tongue with yellow fur, wiry and rapid pulse.

Also indicated for cases of earache accompanied

with irritability, insomnia, red tongue with yellow fur, wiry and strong pulse, which are attributive to adverse rising of liver-fire and dysfunction of orifices.

Also applicable to cases of acute conjunctivitis, scleritis, electric ophthalmia, etc. marked by redness of eyes; cases of glaucoma, hypertension, etc. marked by headache; cases of otitis media, external auditory canal furuncle, etc. marked by earache, which are attributive to stagnation or adverse rising of live-fire.

INTERPRETATION Gentianae is superior for clearing away the sthenic fire from the liver and gall-bladder. Rhei and Gardeniae are helpful to enhance the effect of Gentianae and also can clear away heat through defecation and urination. Ligustici Chuanxiong, Notopterygii and Ledebouriellae are applied for dispersing the stagnated fire. Since the yin-blood is liable to be consumed by the hyperactive live-fire, Angelicae Sinensis is applied to nourish blood and activate blood circulation and is also helpful to enhance the effect of Ligustici Chuanxiong. The acrid-warm nature of Angelicae Sinensis is counteracted by Rhei, and the effect and the effect of activating blood circulation is enhanced when they are used together. Lophatheri has the effects of clearing away heat and relieving listless-

296

ness.

Pill of Cuscutae
(Tu si zi wan)

INGREDIENTS

Semen Cuscutae 15g

Herba Cistanchis 15g

Cornu Cervi Pantotrichum (ground into powder then mixed with decoction)3g

Fructus Schisandrae 6g

Endothelium Corneum Gigeriae Galli 6g

Fructus Alpiniae Oxyphyllae 6g

Radix Linderae 6g

Concha Ostreae Usta 25g

Radix Aconiti Praeparata 10g

Oötheca Mantidis 10g

Rhizoma Dioscoreae 10g

EFFECACY Warming and invigorating kidney-energy and preserving fluid; mainly for cases attributive to insufficiency of kidney-energy and failure of controlling fluid, which are manifested as polyuria, dripping urination, listlessness, intolerance of cold, general debility, dizziness, lumbago, weakness of lower limbs, pale tingue, sunken and weak pulse.

INDICATION 1. For cases of impotence accompanied with dizziness, spiritlessness, lumbago, weakness of lower limbs, sunken and weak pulse, which are attributive to declination of kidney-yang and insufficiency of kidney-yin, omit Concha ostreae and Oötheca and Mantidis from the prescription.

2. Also indicated for cases attributive to deficiency of kidney-energy, which are manifested as frequent nocturnal emission, tinnitus, spiritlessness, fatigue, pale tongue with whitish fur sunken and weak pulse over the chi region.

3. Also applicable to diabetes insipidus, diabeted mellitus, hypertensive renal disease, chronic renal tubular dysfunction, chronic nephritis, etc. marked by polyuria.

INTERPRETATION Cornu Cervi Pantotrichum has the effects of enriching kidney-yang and promoting the production of essential substance, so as to strengthen the muscles and bones. Cuscutae and Cistanchi can tonify kidney-essence and Kidney-yang. Aconiti Praeparata can warm and strengthen kidney-yang. A combination of the above drugs can greatly enrich kidney-energy, and the dripping urination can be controlled. Schisandrae, Oŏtheca Mantidis, Alpiniae Oxypyllae and Usta Concha Ostreae are used for decreasing the amount of urine. Linderae can restore the function of urinary bladder. Endothelium Corneum Gigeriae Galli helps to control urination. Dioscoreae is applied for nourishing spleen-yin.

Powder of Angelicae
Sinensis and Paeoniae
(Dang gui shao yao san)

INGREDIENTS
Radix Angelicae Sinensis 9g
Radix Paeoniae Alba 15g
Rhizoma Ligustici Chuanxiong 6g
Rhizoma Alismatis 10g
Rhizoma Atractylodis Macrocephalae 10g
Poria 12g
EFFICACY Enriching blood, regulating the liver, strengthening the spleen and eliminating dampness; mainly for cases with abdominal pain during pregnancy which can be relieved by pressure, dizziness, oliguria,

edema of feet, light red tongue with white and greasy fur, solf-floating, small and slow pulse, which are attributive to hypofunction of liver and spleen with stagnation of blood and dampness.

INDICATION 1. Applicable to cases of irregular menstruation accompanied with fullness over the lower abdomen, oliguria, puffiness of the face, white and greasy fur on the tongue, wiry and small pulse, which are attributive to hypofunction of liver with blood stagnation and hypofunction of spleen with stagnation of dampness.

2. Also indicated for abdominal mass which is localized and hard, with pain and tenderness, dimmish complexion, thirst without desire to drink, petechiae on the margin of tongue, white and greasy fur on the tongue, wiry and unsmooth pulse, which is attributive to blood stasis and stagnation of dampness.

3. Also applicable to cases of threatened abortion, functional menorrhalgia, premenstrual syndrome, etc. with abdominal pain attributive to hypofunction of liver and spleen and stagnation of blood and dampness; to cases of chronic hepatitis, chronic cholecystitis, early stage of cirrhosis, etc. with abdominal mass attributive to blood stasis and stagnation of dampness.

4. Also appilicable to cases of hypertension, which is attributive to blood-deficiency.

INTERPRETATION Angelicae Sinensis, Paeoniae Alba and Ligustici Chuanxiong have the effects of nourishing blood to regulate the function of the liver and promoting blood circulation and digestion. Atractylodis Macrocephalae, Poria and Alismatis can invigorate the spleen and eliminate dampness. Although Angelicae Sinensis and Ligustici Chuanxiong have a dispersing effect, they can tonify blood without stagnation and promote blood circulation without extravasation when combine with Paeoniae Alba, Alismatis and Poria can strengthen the spleen without causing its stagnation and promote diuresis without causing purgation when combine with Atractylodis Macrocephalae. Moreover, Paeoniae Albe not only can nourish the blood to harmonize yin-energy, but also can nourish the liver to relieve pain. It is particularly indicated for abdominal pain due to hypofunction of the liver with blood stagnation, incoordination between the liver and spleen, and it is used in a larger dose. This prescription is especially applied for pregnant women.

Powder of Ledebouriellae for Dispersing the Superficies
(Fang feng tong sheng San)

INGREDIENTS

Radix Ledebouriellae 10g

Fructus Forsythiae 10g

Fructus Gardeniae 10g

Herba Schizonepetae 6g

Herba Ephedrae 6g

Rhizoma Ligustici Chuanxiong 6g

Radix Angelicae Sinensis 6g

Radix Paeoniae Alba(fried) 6g

Rhizoma Atractylodis Macrocephalae 6g

Radix et Rhizoma Rhei(steamed with wine) 6g

Natrii Sulfas(mixed)6g

Radix Scutellariae 6g

Talcum 20g

Gypsum Fibrosum 15g

Herba Menthae (decocted later) 3g

Radix Platycodi 3g

Radix Glycyrrhizae 3g

Rhizoma Zingiberis Recens 3Pcs

EFFICACY AND INDICATIONS Expelling wind from the body surface, clearing away heat and promoting bowel movement; mainly for sthenia-syndrome of both the superficies and the interior after the attack of exogenous wind-heat and the retention of heat in the interior, which is manifested as aversion to cold fever, dizziness, bitter and dry mouth, conjunctivitis, sorethroat, feeling of oppression over the chest, constipation, dysuria with reddish urine, red tongue with white or yellow fur, floating and smooth, rapid pulse.

1. Applicable to cases of early stage of superficial pyogenic infection with local signs of inflammation, chilliness, fever, bitter mouth, constipation, oliguria, red tongue with white fur, floating and rapid pulse.

2. Also indicated for cases of urticaria and eczema with thin and white fur on the tongue, floating and rapid pulse, which are attributive to simultaneous existence of sthenia-syndrome in the superficies and the interior.

3. Also applicable to cases of influenza, poliomyelitis, infectious mononucleosis, mumps, acute cellulitis, erysipelas, acute lymphangitis, etc., which are attributive to simultaneous existence of sthenia-syndrome in the superficies and the interior after attack of

exogenous wind-heat and retention of heat in the body.

INTERPRETATION

Ledebouriellae, Schizonepetae, Ephedrae, Zingiberis Recens and Menthae serve to expel wind by sweating. Rhei and Natrii Sulfas eliminate the internal heat by purgation, and Gardeniae and Talcum clear away heat by diuresis. Platycodi, Gypsum Fibrosum, Scutellariae and Forsythiae can clear away heat from the lung and stomach. All the above drugs act together to eliminate heat from the upper and the lower part of the body, and treat both the superficies and the interior syndrome. Angelicae Sinensis, Ligustici Chuanxiong and Paeoniae Alba heve the effects of expelling wind and nourishing blood, and Atractylodis Macrocephalae and Glycyrrhizae serve to strengthen the spleen and regulating the stomach; they cooperate each other to exert a diaphoretic effect without damaging the superficies, and exert a purgative effect without impairing the interior. In sum this prescription involves the therapeutic principles of diaphoretic, heat-eliminating, purgative and tonifying simultaneously, aiming at clearing away the internal heat chiefly. The application of Natrii Sulfas and Rhei is for purging heat.

Powder of Peel of Five Drugs
(Wu pi san)

INGREDIENTS

Cortex Zingiberis 9g

Cortex Mori Radicis 9g

Pericarpium Citri Reticulatae 9g

Pericarpium Arecae 9g

Coxtex Poria 9g

EFFICACY AND INDICATIONS Removing dampness to alleviate edema, regulating the flow of qi to strengthen the spleen.

Severe edema due to hypofunction of the spleen with excessive dampness, marked by general dropsy, heavy sensation of the limbs the whole body, distention and fullness in the chest and abdomen, dyspnea, oliguria and edema during pregnency, white and greasy fur of the tongue and deep and slow pulse.

Edema of abrupt onset, edema during pregnancy, and the initial stage of acute nephritis manifested as syndrome of excessive dampness due to hypofunction of the spleen can be treated by the modified recipe.

INTERPRETATION Poria peel in the recipe induce diuresis and excretes dampness, and strengthens the spleen to promote its transporting and transforming water and nutrients at the same time. Ginger Peel, pungent in flavor, disperses fluid-retention. Mulberry bark clears away and purges the lung-qi to dredge water passage. Shell of areca promotes the flow of qi and water to relieve distention and fullness in the abdomen. Tangerine Peel regulates the stomach-qi and resolves turbid dampness. The combined use of the fove drugs produces the effect of inducing diuresis to alleviate edema.

Modern researches have proved that the recipe has the effects of inducing diuresis, regulating intestinal peristalsis, promoting excretion of digestive juice, inducing prespiration and lowering high blood pressure.

CAUTIONS The recipe tends to induce diuresis to alleviate edema, patients with obvious edema due to excessive deficiency of the spleen or accompanied by wind pathogen should be treated by modifying the original recipe.

Prescription for
Treating Hemoptysis
(Ke xue fang)

INGREDIENTS

Indigo Naturalis(dissolved)6g

Semen Trichosanthis 12g

Pumex 12g

Fructus Gardeniae 9g

Fructus Chebulae 6g

Mel q. s.

Succus Zingiberis Recens q. s.

EFFICACY Cooling the liver, stopping bleeding, dispersing phlegm and relieving cough; mainly for cases with hemoptysis attributive to attack of live-fire to the lung, which are manifested as cough, difficult expectoration of thick and bloody sputum, vexation, thirst, flushed cheeks, constipation, yellow fur on the tongue, wiry and rapid pulse.

INDICATION CLINICAL APPLICATION 1. Applicable to cases of rosacea accompanied with irritability, yellow fur, wiry and rapid pulse, which are attributive to attack of the lung by liver-fire and upward attack of lung-heat.

2. For cases of retrograde menstruation manifested as epistaxis during menstruation, non-productive cough, headache, dizziness, congestion of the conjunctiva, red tongue, wiry and rapid pulse, which are attributive to attack of the lung by liver-fire and abnormal rising of blood, omit Chebulae, Pumex and add Herba Artemisiae Annuae and Cortex Moutan Radicis.

3. Also applicable to cases of bronchiectasis, pulmonary tuberculosis, pulmonary hypertension, etc. with hemoptysis, which are attributive to damage of the lung by liver-fire; or cases of hypertension and substitutive menstruation with epistaxis, which are attributed to hyperactivity of liver-fire and abnormal rising of blood.

INTERPRETATION Indigo Naturalis is applied for cleating away sthenic heat from the liver channel, cooling blood and stopping bleeding. Gardeniae has the effects of clearing away heart-fire, calming blood flow, and helps Indigo Naturalis to clear away fire stognated in the liver channel. Pumex and Trichosanthis clear away lung-heat, disperse phlegm, moisten the lung and relieve cough. Semen Trichosanthis acting with Mel can lubricate the intestines and promote bowel

308

movement. Pumex and Succus Zingiberis used together can enhance the expectorant effect. Chebulae serves to astringe the lung-energy, and also enhance the antitussive effec of the above drugs. in sum, this prescription aims chiefly at clearing away liver-fire, so as to ease the lung and stop hemoptysis.

Tablet for Coronary Heart Disease and Hypertension
(Xin xue ning pian)

INGREDIENTS

Pueraria root (Radix Puerariae).

Hawthorn fruit (Fructus Crataegi).

Tablets, 0. 2g each tablet, 100 tablets per bottle.

EFFICACY Dilating coronary artery, increasing the amount of blood flow in coronary artery and cerebral artery, reducing blood-lipid, strengthening cardiac contractility, lowering blood pressure.

INDICATIONS Neck rigidity, dizziness, tinnitus, numbness in limbs and others caused by coronary atherosclerotic cardiopathy, high blood-lipid, and hypertension.

DIRECTION To be taken orally, 3 tablets each time, 3 times a day, or follow the doctor's advice.

Yougui Bolus
(You gui wan)

INGREDIENT
Radix Rehmanniae Praeparata
Rhizoma Dioscoreae
Fructus Corni
Cortex Eucommiae
Fructus Lycii
Radix Aconiti Praeparata
Cortex Cinnamoni
Semen Cuscutae
Radix Angelicae Sinensis
Colla Cornus Cervi
Honeyed Boluses, 9g each bolue.

EFFICACY Warming and invigorating kidney-yang; mainly for cases attributive to insufficiency of kidney-yang, manifested as lumbago, cold limbs, shortness of breath, fatigue, impotence, nocturnal e-mission, pale tongue, small pulse, etc. The action is similar to Yougui Decoction, but its effect is milder and slower, since it is prepared as bolus.

INDICATION Similar as Yougui Decoction.

DIRECTION 9g Tid.

Yougui Decoction
(You gui yin)

INGREDIENTS

Radix Rehmanniae Praeparata 30g

Rhizoma Dioscoreae 10g

Fructus Corni 10g

Cortex Eucommiae 10g

Fructus Lycii 10g

Radix Aconiti Praeparata 7g

Cortex Cinnamomi 3g

Radix Glycyrrhizae Praeparata 3g

EFFICACY Warming and invigorating kidney-yang; mainly for cases attributive to insufficiency of kidney-yang, manifested as lumbago, cold limbs, shortness of breath, fatigue, impotence, nocturnal e-mission, pale tongue, small pulse, etc.

INDICATION 1. The chief action of this prescription is to warm and invigorate kidney-yang, for cases accompanied with deficiency of spleen-yang, manifested as loose stools, poor appetite or vomiting, add Rhizoma Zingiberis; while for cases accompanied with deficiency of spleen-energy, manifested as shortness of breath and fatigue, add Radix Codonopsis pilosulae.

2. For cases of leucorrhagia with thin discharge attributive to insufficiency of kidney-yang, omit Glycyrrhizae and add Semen Cuscutae to tonify the liver and kidney and benefit essence substance.

3. Also applicable to cases of Addison's disease, Sheehan's disease, hypothyroidism, neurasthenia, etc., which are attributive to insufficiency of kidney-yang.

4. Also applicable to case of hypertension, which is manifested as deficiency of both yin and yang.

INTERPRETATION Rehmanniae Praeparata, Corni and Dioscoreae are used for tonifying three yin. Aconiti Praeparata and Cinnamomi are used for warming and tonifying kidney—yang. These yive drugs Supplement each other ane serve as the important drugs for deficiency of kidney-yang. Such a method of composition is actually originated from the Pill for Invigorating

312

Kidney Energy . The Pill for Invigorating Kidney Energy is applied for deficiency of kidney-yang with over-abundance of turbid yin, so that Alismatis and Poria are used together with Aconiti Praeparata to promote diuresis. While this prescription is applied for deficiency of kidney-yang with only small amount of turbid water, so promotion of diuresis is not necessary. Eucommiae and Lycii are used for strengthening tendons and muscles and nourishing liver-blood. Glycyrrhizae Praeparata helps Dioscoreae to benefit middle jiao and nourish the spleen.

Zhenwu Decoction
（Zhen wu tang）

INGREDIENTS
Poria 20g
Radix Paeoniae Alba 20g
Rhizoma Zingiberis Recens 20g
Rhizoma Atractylodis Macrocephalae 10g
Radix Aconiti Praeparata 10g
EFFICACY Warming kidney-yang and promoting diuresis; mainly for cases attributive to exhaustion of

kidney-yang and retention of dampness evil, manifested as dysuria, general edema, or pain and heavy sensation of limbs, or diarrhea.

INDICATIONS 1. For cases of arthritis of cold-dampness type manifested as swelling and pain of the affected joints without redness, which is aggravated by low temperature, add Ramulus Cinnamomi to expel clod evil and relieve pain.

2. For cases of leukorrhagia with thin discharge, attributive to the attack of cold-dampness evil to lower jiao, omit Zingiberis Recens and add Pulvis of Cornu Cervi to warm the kidney and relieve leukorrhagia.

3. Also applicable to cases of renal edema, cardiac edeina aldosteronism, hypertrophy of prostate, hypothyroidism, etc., which are attributive to exhaustion of kidney-yang and retention of dampnes evil.

4. Also applicable to cases of hypertension, which is attributive to asthenia-syndrome.

INTERPRETATION Aconiti has the effects of warming and invigorating spleen-yang and promoting diuresis. Poria and Atractylodis Macrocephalae are used to strengthen the spleen and eliminate dampness. Paeoniae Alba helps Poria to promote diuresis. Zingiberis Recens can disperse dampness and also help Aconiti to warm the tang-energy. This prescription treats edema by regulating the function of spleen and kidney and not by applying diuretics.

Zuogui Decoction
(Zuo gui yin)

INGREDIENTS

Radix Rehmanniae Praeparata 20g

Fructus Corni 10g

Rhizoma Dioscoreae 10g

Fructus Lycii 10g

Poria 6g

Radix Glycyrrhizae Praeparata 3g

EFFICACY Nourishing kidney-yin; mainly for cases attributive to insufficiency of kidney-yin, manifested as lumbago, nocturnal emission, night sweat, dry throat, dizziness, reddish tongue, slow and rapid pulse.

INDICATIONS 1. The chief action of this prescription is to nourish kidney-yin, for cases with dry throat attributive to the inability to generate each other between the lung and the kidney, add Radix Ophiopogonis to nourish lung-yin; for cases with hectic fever and profuse sweating attributive to yin-deficiency and fire hyperactivity, add Cortex Lycii Radicis to clear away the asthenic heat.

2. Also applicable to cases of tuberculosis, hypertension, hypothyroidism, Addison's disease, etc. which are attributive to insufficiency of kidney-yin but without hyperactivity of fire.

INTERPRETATION Rehmanniae Praeparata tonifies kidney-yin, Corni nourishes liver-yin, and Dioscoreae invigorates spleen-yin. This prescription tonifies three yin at the same time, similar to the Bolus of Six Drugs Containing Rehmanniae Praeparata. But the later deals with the cases with deficiency of yin and hyperactivity of fire, while the Zuogui Decoction is indicated for yin-deficiency cases without hyperactivity of fire. So Lycii is applied in the prescription for tonifying yin-blood, and a small dose of Poria and Glycyrrhizae Praeparata for strengthening the spleen and benefiting vital energy.

Chapter Five
ACUPUNCTURE TREATMENT

1 Body acupuncture:

1) For excess of liver-fire: Quchi(LI 11)、Tai-chong(LR 3)、Fengchi(GB20)、Taiyang(EX-HN 5). Manipulated with reducing or even movement method.

2) For excess of phlegm-dampness: Quchi (LI 11)、Taichong(LR 3)、Fenglong(ST 40)、Zhongwan (RN 12)、Neiguan(PC 6). Manipulated with reducing or even movement method.

3) For hyperactivity of yang due to yin deficiency: Quchi(LI 11)、Taichong(LR 3)、Shenshu(BL 23)、Ganshu(BL 18)、Taixi(KI 3)、Sanyinjiao(SP 6). Manipulated with reinforcing method.

4) Points used to calm liver yang: Fengchi(GB 20)、Baihui(DU 20)、Xuanlu(GB 5)、Xiaxi(GB 43) Xingjian (LR 2). Manipulated with the reducing method.

5) Points to replenish and regulate qi and blood: Baihui(DU 20)、Qihai(RN 6)、Ganshu(BL 18)、Pishu(BL 20)、Shenshu(BL 23)、Zusanli(ST 36), manipulated with the reinforcing method.

6) Points to tonify the kidneys: Baihui (DU 20),
Shenshu (BL 23), Sanyinjiao (SP 6), Fengchi (GB
20), Qihai (RN 6), Taixi (KI 13), Guanyuan (RN 4).
Manipulated with the reinforcing method.

7) Points to resolve phlegm and eliminate damp:
Baihui (DU 20), Fengchi (GB 20), Touwei (ST 8),
Pishu (BL 20), Zhongwan (RN 12), Neijuan (PC 6),
Fenglong (ST 40). Manipulated with the reducing
method.

8) Points: Quchi (LI 11), Fengchi (GB 20),
Tianzhu (BL 10), Zusanli (ST 36), Taichong (LR 3),
Hegu (LI 4), Taiyang (EX-HN 5).

Method: Puncture from Qichi (LI 11) towards
Shaohae (HT 3), deep insertion is done in Tianzhu (BL
10) for 1—1.5cun. There is no letention of needles.
Or singly puncture Quchi (LI 11) with the reducing
method of lifting, thrusting and rotating the needle.
Blood pressure may be lower 30 minutes after acupuncture.

Headache, dizziness and distension of head:
Taiyang (EX-HN 5), Fengchi (GB 20), Yintang (EX-
HN 3), Hegu (LI 4), Taichong (LR 3).

Tinnitus: Waiguan (SJ 5), Yifeng (SJ 17).

Insomnia: Shenmen (HT 7), Sanyinjiao (SP 6).

Palpitation: Neiguan(PC 6), Ximen(PC 4).

Anorexia: Zusanli(ST 36).

Excessive phlegm: Fenglong (ST 40), Zhongwan (RN 12).

9) Main Points: Quchi (LI 11)Zhsanli (ST 36)、Fengchi(GB 20)、Taichong(LR 3).

Complementary points: Add Yintang (EX-HN3)、Taiyang(EX-HN5)for headache; add Sanyinjiao (SP 6)、Shenmen (HT 7) for insomnia; add Ximen(PC4)、Neiguan (PC6)for palpitation.

Method: The two groups and used alternatively once a day or every other day. 10 treatments make a course. Use the filiform needles to puncture the points with reducing method for excessive syndrome, with reinforcing method for deficient syndrome, with even manipulation for deficiency in origin and excess in the superficiality.

2. Ear acupuncture

1) Prescription: Kidney, Adrenal Gland, Infraantihelix Crus End, Brain and Ear-shenmen.

Method: Select 2 — 3 points in each treatment. Puncture the points with moderate or strong stimulation. Retain the needles for 20 to 30 minutes and manipulate the needles intermittently.

319

2) Prescription: Pt. Heart, Pt. Liver, Pt. Middle Border. Pt. Groove for Lowering Blood Pressure, Pt. Shenmen and Pt. Ear Apex.

Methos: 3 — 5 points are selected for each treatment. A moderate or strong stimulation is given. Retain the needles for 1 — 2 hours. Give the treatment once each day. Pt. Groove for Lowering Blood Pressure may be pricked to cause bleeding with a three-edged needle. The disease may be treated by auricular-seed-pressing therapy.

3. Scalp acupuncture

Prescription: Foot motor sensory area (bilateral), Thoracic area, and Vasomotor area.

Method: Give the treatment once each day. 5 — 10 treatments make up a course.

Chapter Six

MASSAGE FOR HYPERTENSION TREATMENT

1. Prescription and Symptomatic Point Selection

Press-knead Baihui (DU 20), Yintang (EX-HN3), Taiyang (EX-HN5) and Fengchi (GB 20) 30 times each, push Qiaogong 30 times, rub Shenque (RN 8) 30 times, scrub the hypochondria (both sides) 30 times, thump Jianjing (GB 2) 30 times, pat the upper back 30 times, and press-knead Neiguan (PC 6), Quchi (LI 11), Zusanil (ST 36) and Sanyinjiao (SP 6) 30 times cach.

Hypertensive patients with severe headache may conduct massage by modifying the prescription for headache.

Hypertensive patients with vetigo and tinnitus, vexation and amnesia and soreness and weakness of the loins and knees may, additionally, press-knead Fengfu (DU 16), Tinghui (GB 2), Shenshu (BL 23) and Zhishi (BL 52) 30 times each, Scrub Yaoyan (the small of back) 30 times, and nip-knead Taixi(KI 3) and Taichong (LR 3) 30 times each.

Hypertensives with headache and severe dizziness, vertigo, nausea, and stuffiness and distension in the chest and epigastric region accompanied with poor appetite should add the following manipulations: rubbing Zhongwan (RN 17) 30 times, and press-kneading Pishu (BL 20) and Weishu (BL 21) 30 times each.

Hypertensive patients with stuffiness and pain in the chest, palpitation, insomnia and dreaminess should, additionally, knead Xinshu (BL 15) 30 times, push-scrub the prothorax 30 times, and press-knead Tanzhong (RN 17), Rugen(ST 18), Shenshu (BL 23) and Yongquan(K 1) 30 times each.

2. The second method

Press-knead Baihui (DU 20), Yintang (EX-HN3), Taiyang (EX-HN5), Fengchi(GB 20), Fengfu (DU 16), Tinghui (GB2), Shenshu (BL 23), Zhishi(BL 52), Pishu (BL 20), Weishu (BL 21), and Xinshu (BL 15),for 30 times respectively. Push Qiaogong for 30 times. Rub Shenque (RN 8) and Zhongwan (DU 12) for 30 times respectively. Chafe the both hypochondria and Yaoyan (EX-B7)for 30 times respectively. Thump Jianjing (GB 21) for times. Pat the upper back for 30 times. Nip-knead Taixi(KI 3)and Tai-chong (LR 3) for 30 times respectively, and press-knead Neiguan(PC 6),Quchi(LI 11), Zhsanli(ST 36) and Sanyinjiao (SP 6) for 30 times respectively. Knead Danzhong(RN 17) for 30 times.

3. The third method

This massage therapy is mainly curative for benigh hypertension to remit the various Symptoms, especially for primary hypertension if there is a constant therapy, in such case, by function of nerve reflex and humoral regulation, the inhibited activites of cerebral cortex can be increased to regulate the function of vasomotor cen-ter, bringing about hypotension and blood pressure de-creasing of small arteries. Subsequently the symptoms may remit or disappear.

1) Manipulation: Pushing with one-finger medita-tion, lifting-grasping, pressing-kneading, arching-pushing with elbow and rubbing.

2) Location of Points: Fengchi(GB 20), Dazhui (DU 14),Huantiao(GB30), Baihui(DU 20) and Qiao-gong.

3) Operation

(1) Standing behind the patint, the doctor lift-grasps the cervical portion for 30-50 times.

（2）With the mainipulation of thumb-straight-pushing, the doctor pushes the left and right Qiaogong from above to below for 30-50 times each side.

（3）With the manipulation of one-finger pushing, the doctor repeatedly and alternatively pushes from Yintang (EX-HN 3), by way of superciliary arch, to Taiyang (EX-HN 5), then to Touwei (ST 8), Shuaigu (GB 8), Fubai (GB 10) and Naokong (GB 19), for 3-5 minutes.

（4）With the thumb and the four fingers, the doctor grasps from the front the head, along the channels of DU, Shaoyang and Taiyang, to the back of the head for 3-5 times.

（5）With the manipulation of one-finger pushing, the doctor pushes Dazhui(DU 14) for 3-5 minutes.

（6）The doctor sits to the right of the patient who is in a supine position, and rubs the abdomen clockwise for 5-7 minutes.

（7）The patient in lateral-lying posision, the doctor elbow-motions Huantiao (GB 30) for 5 — 7 minutes.

（8）The patient is in a prone position, with the waist and sacrum coated with Chinese holly leaf ointment. With minor thenar eminance the doctor horizontally-Scrubs the waist and sacrum till they become penetratedly hot.

(9) With the thumb, the doctor pushes Yongquan (KI 1) for 3-5 minutes.

4) Course of Treatment: Once a day, 10 times as one course; with an interval of 2 or 3 days between two courses.

Chapter Seven

QIGONG TREATMENT OF HYPERTENSION

1. Self-Treatment by Practising Qigong

1) Basic Maneuvers

It is advisable to practise Relaxation Qigong, Head and Face Qigong, Neck and Nape Qigong, Upper Limbs Qigong and Lower Limbs Qigong.

2) Auxiliary Maneuvers

(1) Hyperactivity of yang due to yin deficiency: It is advisable to practise Gathering Moon Cream Qigong.

(2) Flaring liver-fire: It is advisable to practise

the methods of rubbing the chest and training qi with the work "xu" as well as soothing the liver and conductiong qi in Regulating Liver Qigong.

(3) Deficiency of both yin and yang: It is advisable to practise the method of taking black qi in Regulating-kidney Qigong and the method of taking yellow qi in Regulating-splen Qigong, or practise Gathering Sun Essence and Moon Cream Qigong.

2. External Qi (Waiqi) Therapy

1) Basic Maneuvers

(1) Push and smear Yintang (Glabella, Ex-HN3) and Kangong (North Palace, 1 cun over the eyebrow and directly above the pupil), sweep Shuaigu (Following the Valley, GB 8) and Hanyan (Disgust with Nodding, GB 4) with the fingers in a combing way, press and knead Baihui (Hundred Convergences, DU 20), Fengchi (Wind Pond, GB 20) and Dazhui (Big Vertebra, DU 14).

(2) Apply the flat-palm form, use the vibrating and quivering manipulations to emit qi onto Baihui (Hundred Convergences, DU 20), Dazhui (Big Vertebra, DU 14), Mingmen (Gate of Life, DU 4) and Zhongwan (Middle Epingastrium, RN 12) for 6 or 16 breaths respectively, then apply the middlefinger

standing-alone form, use the vibrating and quivering manipulations to emit qi onto Zhongwan (Middle Epigastrium, RN 12) and Guanyuan (Energy Pass, RN 4) for 6 or 12 breaths.

(3) apply the flat-palm form, use the pulling and leading manipulations to emit qi onto Baihui (Hundred Convergences, DU 20) and Touwei (Head Corner, ST 8), and conduct qi downward along the DU Channel and the STomach Channel to cause qi to be void in the upper part and replete in the lower part.

2) Auxiliary Maneuvers

(1) Hyperactivity of yang due to yin deficiency: Apply the flat-palm form, use the pushing and rotating manipulations to emit qi onto Ganshu (Liver Shu, BL 18), Shenshu (Kidney Shu, BL 23) and Dantian (Elixir Field), and use the rightward-rotating maneuver to conduct qi along the channel.

(2) Flaring liver-fire: apply the flat-palm form, use the pulling and leading manipulations to emit qi onto the acupoint of Zhangmen (Bright Door, LR 13), Qimen (Cyclic Door, LR 14) and Riyue (Sun and Moon, GB 24), and conduct qi along the LRer Channel and the Gallbladder Channel to the lower limbs.

(3) Deficiency of both yin and yang: Apply the

flat-palm form, use the rightward-rotating manipulation to emit qi onto Pishu(Spleen Shu, BL 20),Shenshu (Kidney Shu, BL 23), Mingmen(gate of Life, DU 4) and Dantian(Elixir Field).

3. The Third Method

The tongue tip touches the hard palate. the eyes Slightly droop. the chest slightly draws in and the back erects. Regulate breathing and concentrate the mind on Dantian. Then regard the whole body as a point to relax. Read silently to effect a general one-shot relaxation from the head to the feet; or silently meditate to fly and fall from a high place to relax.

4. The Fourth Method

Assume the standing or sitting posture. Place both palms flatly on both hypochondria and inhale slowly. When exhaling, utter the "xu"word-formula. Meanwhile, gently rub both costal regions in circular motion with both palm. Do 10 or breaths.

Qigong (breathing exercise) therapy has also shown promise in relieving hypertension. One study randomly divided 204 patients with esential hypertension into two group: 104 cases received Qigong therapy plus a small amount of hypotensor and 100 cases in the control group recrived a small amount of western hypotensor only. Two months after treatment the hypotensive effect rate was 91 percent both in Qigong group and in the control group. Twenty years later it was 88 percent in the Qigong group and 67 percent in the control group. DUring the 20 years doctors followed the progess of these patients, they found that the incidence of stroke and the rate of mortality were 16. 35 persent and 11. 54 percent, respectively, in the Qigong group, and 30 percent and 23 percent, respectively, in the control group. These studies showed that Qigong played a major role in improving the self-regulation function and in relieving multiple cerebro-cardiovascular risk factors.

Chapter Eight
MEDICATED DIET TREATMENT
FOR HYPERTENSION

Medicated diet can be used not only as a supplementary treatment for essential hypertension but also for its prevention and recovery and for health care.

1. Food for Treating Hypertension

1) Hawthorn fruit (Fructus Crataegi) The drug has the function of bringing down blood pressure and is to be taken 9 to 15g per day. It is applcable to patients with essential hypertension or that accompanied with hyperlipemia and coronary heart disease.

2) Chrysanthemum flower (Flos Chrysanthemi) It can bring down blood pressur and can be taken as a drink for a long time, 6 to 12g per day. This drug is applicable to essential hypertension marked by the types of flaming-up of liver-fire or of hyperactivity of yang due to yin deficiency.

3) Celery (Apium) It contains apin which functions in bringing down blood pressur. Cut up 250g of fresh celery and extract its juice, which is to be taken twice a day. Or decoct not for long 30 to 60g of fresh

celery for oral administration. This drug is applicable to essential hypertension manifestd as the type of flaming-up of liver-fire or hyperactivity of yang due to yin deficiency.

4) Onilon (Bulbus Allii cepae) Having the function of promoting digestion, onion can prevent and treat hypertension. It can be either pounded to get its juice for drinking or eaten sauteed.

5) Garlic (Bulbus Allii) Garlic contains allin that can bring down blood pressure and is to be eaten raw, stewed, or cooked in gruel. It can be decocted, or pounded and made into boluses or pills for oral administration.

6) Carrot (Radix Dauci Carotae) It can be eaten raw or cooked, or be decocted, or extracted to get its juice for oral administration.

7) Shepherd's purse (Herba Capsellae) Fresh shepherd's purse is to be extracted to get its juice, or decocted, for oral administration. It can be eaten stir-fried, too. It is applicable to essential hypertension marked by the type of flaming-up of liver-fire. The common dosage is 30 to 60g each time.

8) Japanese sea tangle (Thallus Eckloniae) The laminine, the drug contains, can bring down blood

pressure. Usually it is to be taken 15 to 60g per day. It can be eaten cooked, or decocted for oral administration, or used as an ingredient of boluses or pills or powder.

9) Straw mushroom (Volva Fungorum) Fresh straw mushroom should be eaten boiled or stir-fried. The common dosage is 30 to 60g each time.

10) Miscellanies tremella (Tremella), jew's ear (Auricularia), wild rice shoots (Rhizoma Zizaniae), apple (Malum Silvestre), pear (Malum Piri), persimmon (Fructus Kaki) and tangerine (Fructus Citri Tangerinae) can be selected for eating. In addition, corn stigma (STigma Maydis) decoction, when taken orally, can also bring down blood presure and induce diuresis.

2. Composite Medicated Diet

1) Drink of Hawthorn Fruit and Chrysanthemum Flower (Shanzha Juhua Daichayin)

INGREDIENTS

Fructus Crataegi 12g

Flos Chrysanthemi 9g

PROCESS Infuse above foods in boiling water for drinking.

DIRECTIONS Patients with essential hypertension or accompanied with hyperlipemia, coronary heart disease can take it regularly as tea; while those with essential hypertension marked by the types of liver-fire or hyperactivity of yang due to yin deficiency can take it as a supplementary medicine.

2) Thick Soup or Water Chestnut and Jellyfish Head(Xuegeng Tang)

INGREDIENTS

Bulbus Heleocharis Tuberosae 100-200g

Rhopilema 100-200g

PROCESS Cook soup with above foods.

DIRECTIONS To be taken twice or three times a day for the treatment of essential hypertension accompanied with syndrome of accumulation of phlegm manifested clinically as vertigo, heaviness sensation in the head, fullness and stuffiness in the chest and stomach, or vomiting, nausea, salivation, white and greasy fur, wiry and slippery pulse.

3) Soup of Corn Stigma and Tortoise (Yumixu Gui tang)

INGREDIENTS

Chinemys Reevesii(over 500g) 1

Stigma Maydis 120g

PROCESS place the tortoise in a basin, pour in

hot water; after the tortoise has discharged all its urine, wash it clean and cut off its head and feet, rid it of its internal organs; then put it in an earthenware pot together with the corn stigma and a right amount of water. Cook on a strong fire until the water comes to the boil then cook on with a slow fire until the tortoise is well-done.

DIRECTIONS The flesh of the tortoise is for eating and the soup for drinking. It is used to treat essential hypertension manifested as the type of deficiency of both the liver-yin and the kidney-yin.

4) Gruel of Chrysanthemum Flower and Hawthorn Fruit (Juhua Shanzha Zhou)

INGREDIENTS

Flos Chrysanthemi(with no bases) 9—12g

Fructus Crataegi 9—12g

Semen oryzae Sativae 45—60g

crystal sugar right amount

PROCESS Grind the first two ingredients into powder; then make gruel out of the rice, sugar and 500ml of water, when the rice begins to boil with the liquid not thick yet, mix the powder of the first two ingredients into the gruel and go on cooking on a slow fire for a while; and finally when the gruel becomes thick, put out the fire and simmer it for five minutes with the pot tightly covered.

DIRECTIONS To be baken warm, once or twice a day, for patients with esential hypertension or that accompanied with hyperlipemia, coronary heart disease. STop taking it in winter.

5) Decoction of Celery and Chinese-Date (Qincai Dazao Tang)

INGREDIENTS

Herba Apii 60g

Fructus Ziziphi Jujubae 30g

PROCESS Dococt the above drugs in a right amout of water.

DIRECTIONS To be taken twice a day over a month in succession.

6) Decoction of Hawthorn Fruit and Cassia Seed (Shanzha Jueming Tang)

INGREDIENTS

Fructus Crataegi 15—30g

Semen Cassiae 15—30g

PROCESS Dococt them in a right amount of water for oral administration or infuse them in boiling water for drinking.

DIRECTIONS Applicable to patients with both

essential hypertension and hyperlipemia accompanied with constipation. The amount of cassia seed should be reduced when the patient is free from constipation.

7) Drink of Chrysanthemum Flower, sophora Flower and Green Tea (Ju Hua Lucha Yin)

INGREDIENTS

Flos Chrysanthemi 3—6g

Flos Sophorae 3—6g

Folium Camelliae Viride 3g

PROCESS Infuse them in boiling water for drinking.

RIRECTIONS Its indications are the same as those of Drink of Hawthorn Fruit and Chrysanthemum Flower.

8) Soup of Tremella and Jew's Ear (Shuang Er Tang)

INGREDIENTS

Tremella 9—12g

Auricularia 9—12g

crystal sugar right amount

PROCESS First soak the first two ingredients in warm water and wash them clean; then place them in a bowl, pour water into the bowl and add in the crystal sugar; and finally steam them in a food steamer for an hour.

DIRECTIONS The tremella and the jew's eat are for eating and the soup for drinking, once or twice per day. It is applicable to patients with essential hypertension, arteriosclerosis or that accompanied with bleeding from the eyeground, especially good for the type of deficiency of both the liver-yin and the kidney-yin.

9) Soup of Mung Bean and Kelp (Haidai Lüdou Tang)

INGREDIENTS

Semen Phaseoli Radiati 90g

Thallus Laminariae 45g

Crystal sugar right amount

PROCESS Cook the three ingredients together in water over a strong fire until the water comes to the boil; then cook over a slow fire until the mung bean and the kelp are welldone.

DIRECTIONS This soup is for eating. taking it regularly can prevent essential hypertension and hyperlipemia.

Select one or two from among the recipes above that are to your taste. If curative, they should be taken for a long time.

3. The Others

The patient can choose any of the following recipes according to individual conditions.

Frequently eat black edible fungus cooked with scallions and garlic. this can delay the formation of blood clots and reduce the occurrence of arteriosclerosis.

Soak peanuts in vinegar for a week. Eat 10 peanuts morning and evening. This softens blood vessels and reduces blood pressure.

Mix evenly 60g of green bean flour and .20g of pig gall powder. Three gram doses should be taken three times a day. This can lower blood pressure.

Dry edible sea weeds in the sun and grind them into fine powder. Six gram daily, divided into three doses, for one to three months. Edible sea weeds may also be stewed or steamed and eaten at meals. This can reduce blood pressure; prevent and treat cancer of the digestive tract.

Chapter Nine
NURSING OF HPERTENSION DISEASE

1. General Nursing

1) Ward light should not be strong, the environment should be quiet and comfortable, and sleeping time should be assured.

2) The patient with initial hypertension may take part in work, but must not be overtird, and should regularly do exercises such as Taiji quan, Qigong, etc.

3) Diet should be low caloria, light, plenty of vegetables, fruits, high in vitamines and with a litle Salt. Peppery, sweat, fat and greasy food is contraindicated and drinking must be abstained from completely.

4) Watch for changes of blood pressure, if the blood pressure is in obvious undulation, the doctor should be informed in order to take measure.

2. Nursing According to Syndrome Differentiation.

1) Fire-syndrome due to Stagnation of the Liver-qi and Hyperactivity of the liver yang.

Clinical Manifestations

Dizziness, flushed complexion, red eyes, irritability, bitter taste in the mouth, dry throat, scanty and dark urination, reddish tongue, wiry, rapid and forceful pulse.

Nursing

(1) Understand the patient's psychology, give the patient psychological nursing to assist him to free his mind of anxiety and anger, keep ease of mind and optimistic attitude.

(2) The traditional Chinese drugs should be taken to clear and purge liver-heat and assist in nourishing Yin. The selected prescription is Longdan Xiegan Tang with modification(Modified Decoction of Gentiana for Purging the LRer-fire). Longdan Xiegan Wan (Pill to Purge the LRer Fire with Gentiana)9 g is taken each time, twice a day.

(3) Acupuncture an moxibustion.

(4) Flos Chrysanthemi 60g is boiled for oral use instead of tea.

2) Hyperactivity of the Liver-Yang due to Both Deficiency of the Liver-Yin and Kidney-Yin.

Clinical Manifestations

Dizziness, tinnitus, insomnia, frequent dreaming, irritability, difficult and dark urine, lumbago and lassitude in legs, numbness of limbs in the severe case, wiry and thin pulse and dark red tongue.

Nursing

(1) Watch carefully for changes of patient's condition, in the case of symptoms and signs of apoplexy such as numbness of lips and tongue, numbness of extremities, deviation of the eye and mouth, the patient must take immediate bed rest and the doctor should be notified promptly to give treatment.

(2) Since every attack of the disease is due to tiredness or anger, rest and emotional care are essential.

(3) Acupuncture and moxibustion.

(4) Naoliqing 10 — 20 pills is taken each time, twice a day.

(5) The traditional Chinese drugs should be taken to nourish liver-Yin and kidney-yin, tranquilize and subdue hyperactive liver-Yang. The selected prescription is Zhengan Xifeng Tang with modification (Modified Tranquilizing the Liver-wind Decoction). the decoction should be taken warm.

3) Upward Invasion of Yang due to deficiency of Both Yin and Yang

Clinical Manifestations

Headache, dizziness, blurred vision, tinnitus,

light red face, dry mouth, spontaneous-perspiration, insomnia, frequent dreaming, soreness of the loins, cold limbs, muscular twiching and cramp, short breath on exertion, dark red tongue with scanty coating, wiry and thin pulse.

Nursing

(1) Diet should be supervised strictly, Chinese date, sesame seed, Chinses yam, walnut, etc. should be mostly eaten.

(2) The traditional Chinese drugs should be taken for nourishing the kidney-yin, warming the kidney-yang. The selected prescription is Shenqiwan with modification (Modified Bolus for Tonifying the Kidney-Qi). Guifudihuang Wan (Pills of Cinnamon Twig, Prepared Aconite Root and Rehmannia Root) 1 pill is taken each time, twice daily.

(3) Acupuncture and moxibustion treatment.

图书在版编目(CIP)数据

中医治疗高血压病：英文/侯景伦编著；李国华译.-
北京：学苑出版社,1995.9
ISBN 7-5077-0996-5

I.中… II.①侯-②李…中医治疗法-III.高血压-中医治疗法-
英文 IV . R259.441

中国版本图书馆 CIP 数据核字(95)第 16075 号

中医治疗高血压病

主　编　　侯景伦
副主编　　任武贤
编　委　李福林　林　祺　李国华　刘建新

学苑出版社出版
(中国北京万寿路西街 11 号)
邮政编码 100036
北京大兴沙窝店印刷厂印刷
中国国际图书贸易总公司发行
(中国北京车公庄西路 35 号)
北京邮政信箱第 399 号　邮政编码 100044
版次：英文版　32 开本　1995 年 9 月第一版第一次印刷
ISBN7-5077-0996-5/R・165

05950
14-E-2874 P